Children with
ASTHMA
A Manual for Parents

Second edition, completely updated

THOMAS F. PLAUT, M.D.
with parents, patients, and physicians

Pedipress, Inc.
Amherst, Massachusetts

NOTICE

The indications and dosages of all drugs in this book have been recommended in the medical literature and conform to the practice of asthma experts throughout the country. However, the information provided here is general and may not apply to your child's specific situation. DO NOT CHANGE YOUR MEDICATION ROUTINE WITHOUT YOUR DOCTOR'S APPROVAL.

Library of Congress Cataloging-in-Publication Data

Plaut, Thomas F., 1933–
   Children with asthma.

   Bibliography: p.
   Includes index.
   1. Asthma in children. I. Title.
RJ436.A8P56   1988   618.92′238   87–34311
ISBN 0–914625–03–9 (pbk.)

88 89 90 91 92.   10 9 8 7 6 5 4 3 2

Second Edition

Book Design by Robin Brooks and Barbara Werden

*Dedicated to parents, patients, and physicians
who are willing to learn*

Contents

Forms

Tables

Illustrations

About the Author

Thomas F. Plaut, M.D., has practiced pediatrics for over twenty years and has cared for hundreds of children with asthma. The parents of these patients have asked difficult questions and demanded understandable answers. In addition, they have observed their children's daily reaction to asthma and the medications used to treat it. They have taught their pediatrician more about asthma than he ever could have observed in the office.

Plaut graduated from Yale University with a bachelor's degree in history and received his medical degree from Columbia University. After a pediatric residency at New York University-Bellevue Medical Center in New York City, he practiced in Whitesburg, Kentucky, and then spent ten years at the Martin Luther King Health Center in the South Bronx. He joined Amherst Medical Associates in 1977 and founded Asthma Consultants in 1988. He now devotes his full energy to helping families and institutions improve the care of children with asthma.

Plaut believes that almost every parent whose child has asthma has the desire and the ability to manage asthma at home. Many health professionals greatly underestimate this ability. He believes that hospitalization for asthma will be rare once parents learn the basics of home management.

The author has presented his views on asthma to parents, teachers, and the general public at lectures, seminars and on radio and television. He regularly presents his research findings to health professionals in journal articles, workshops, and national meetings.

Preface

Asthma care which was good enough in 1983 when *Children With Asthma* was first published is not good enough today. You and your doctor can now do a much more effective job in preventing and treating asthma episodes.

Though we use many of the same drugs that we used five years ago, we have learned how to balance their good and bad effects much better. We use inhaled drugs—adrenergics, cromolyn, and steroids—much more frequently than in the past. These changes are reflected in the medication chapter and a new chapter on home treatment.

New sections cover the diagnosis of asthma, the early treatment of asthma episodes, and a way to monitor the progress of an asthma episode. Infants and teenagers receive more attention in this edition. We also describe the contributions of family members and support groups to asthma care. Finally, we look in on six children several years after meeting them in the first edition.

Thirty new illustrations portray details of the respiratory system and the asthma process. They also depict the peak flow meters and inhalation devices which are so important in the treatment of asthma today.

The resource and medical reference sections can guide you to additional reading and to organizations which provide information and support to families of children with asthma.

Thomas F. Plaut, M.D.
Amherst, Massachusetts

xix

Acknowledgments

Parents of children with asthma at Amherst Medical Center have been involved in every step of this book's development. They have asked for basic information in a form that they could understand. They have learned about asthma and strongly felt that other parents should be spared the misinformation, inadequate treatment, and lack of support with which they had had to contend. Jeamie Duffy sat down one night, and after writing for six hours, completed "Matthew," the account of her son's first seven years. Reading that account encouraged other parents to write of their experiences. All tell different stories but the message is the same: parents can learn to improve their child's asthma care with the support of their physician.

The entire pediatric staff of the Amherst Medical Center contributed to the evolution of this book by treating our patients with competence, caring and respect. Sally Howland, R.N., Mary Wing, R.N., Martha Barstow, R.N., Shirley Quinlan, R.N., Ingrid Dybvik, R.N., Jackie Gladu, R.N., Audrey Kilcoyne, R.N., Edna McAveney, Norma Hallock, P.N.P., Ruth Sullivan, P.N.P., Anne Gray, Diana Kocot, Lois Kelley, R.N., Mary Dent, R.N., Linda Haney, R.N., Rosemary Koffler, R.N., Cathy Boyd, R.N., Diane Green, Eleanor Boluch, Leslie Champoux, Eva Adamski, Nora Cuddy, Lana King, Linda Reif, and Lori Mruk provided care and created an atmosphere which made it easy for parents to learn about asthma. Beth Gradone assisted me with efficiency and good humor. Health educator, Sharon Dorfman, convinced me that parents need more than facts and skills.

Guillermo Mendoza, M.D., more than any other individual, was a source of information and support. His knowledge of peak flow

xxi

monitoring was invaluable. Thomas Creer, Ph.D., and Guy Parcel, Ph.D., were generous in providing information and encouragement throughout the entire project. Robert Zwerdling, M.D., Paul Walker, M.D., Miles Weinberger, M.D., Jay Selcow, M.D., Nancy Sander, Carlton Palm, M.D., Constantine J. Falliers, M.D., Renee Bergner, M.D., and Arthur Bergner, M.D., provided valuable insights. Karen Emilson Schroeder, Debra Scherrer, Ian Nathanson, M.D., Henry Levison, M.D., Andrew Larkin, M.D., David Jamison, Elliot Ellis, M.D., Georgie Cathey, R.Ph., and Herb Behrens, criticized the manuscript and improved it greatly; any remaining errors are mine. Emlen Jones, M.D., contributed to the sections on cromolyn and judging the severity of an attack and Michael Posner, M.D., contributed to the section on coughing asthma in the first as well as this edition.

My colleagues, David Marsh, M.D., Kathy Chrismer, M.D., Emlen Jones, M.D., David Gottsegen, M.D., Michael Posner, M.D., and Arlen Collins, M.D., shared in the day-to-day care of these patients as did all the family practitioners on the staff of the Amherst Medical Center. I could not have written this book without their support.

Carla Brennan produced the lucid illustrations. Heidi Nordberg and Nancy Newcombe tied up loose ends. Happi Cramer produced the manuscript with good nature and skill.

Finally, I want to thank my son, David, for discussing asthma with me, my daughter, Rebecca, for her help with the first edition, and my wife Johanna for her continuing support. Thanks to the three of you for tolerating the disruption which this book inevitably caused in our family's life.

Children With Asthma

Introduction

Childhood asthma is a chronic illness that affects five to ten percent of the children in the United States. It is frequently misdiagnosed or undertreated and causes more hospital admissions, more visits to hospital emergency rooms and more school absences than any other chronic disease of childhood. When asthma is not well-controlled, it may severely disrupt the living patterns of the families affected by it.

A child with undertreated asthma may experience an episode suddenly and with little warning, causing panic and upheaval in the family unprepared to respond. The seeming unpredictability of asthma episodes may cause parents to worry incessantly and needlessly about their child's well-being. When an asthma episode occurs in school, it causes anxiety for everyone around: the child, the teacher and the nurse. Asthma also interferes with extra-curricular activities. Breathing trouble during a sporting event not only embarrasses the child, but often brings advice to reduce activity. Such restrictions damage the child's self-esteem and are rarely necessary.

Can we improve the ability of parents and their children with asthma to manage asthma at home? The answer is a definite yes.

When you and your physician work together you will almost always be able to develop a comprehensive treatment plan which allows your child to lead a fully active life. You can gain the knowledge, skill, and attitudes essential to improve your child's care. It takes no special ability to learn how asthma affects the lungs and how various aspects of treatment can reverse or prevent an episode. All it takes is the knowledge you can gain from this book and a good amount of practice.

Parents need to learn how to recognize the four signs of asthma trouble and how to keep an asthma diary. You need to learn about each medicine your child takes. You must develop skill in the use of a peak flow meter, a metered-dose inhaler, a holding chamber and a compressor-driven nebulizer as recommended by your physician. You should be able to use these devices easily and with confidence when you need them. In addition, you need to learn what you can handle yourself and when to ask your physician for help.

Because words often guide our attitudes, the language that parents and doctors use about children with asthma is important. The patient is not "an asthmatic." He or she is a child with asthma. Referring to a child as an asthmatic describes the child in terms of the problem and thus distorts the attitudes of parents, physicians, teachers and friends. A child with asthma, on the other hand, is generally healthy but has a problem that requires care. Using the words episode or flare instead of the word attack is also a conscious choice. "Attack" sounds overly dramatic, and well-controlled asthma is not very dramatic.

Goals are also important. With rare exceptions, it should be assumed that every patient will be able to carry out every activity that is usual for his or her age. A child who wants to play hockey, run cross-country, or compete in swimming should be encouraged to do so. Children with asthma can and do take part in all of these activities. Assumptions should not be based on a child's past history. Just because a child has been hospitalized many times for asthma does not mean that the child will require such care after a comprehensive program of treatment has improved control over the asthma problem. Only rarely should it be necessary to ask the school to excuse a child from gym class because of asthma. Almost all children with well-controlled asthma can participate in regular gym activities without restriction.

Ten years ago, there was no satisfactory way to control asthma in a child with mild to moderate disease. The best that a parent could do was to give a combination medication for a mild problem and to take the child to the doctor's office or emergency room for a shot of epinephrine in the case of a more severe episode.

Some recent developments have made asthma a much more manageable illness.

Peak flow meter: Several models are now available for home use at a reasonable price. They measure the flow of air from the child's lung. They can be used to monitor the effectiveness of treatment. They can also give an early warning that an episode is starting.

Inhaled adrenergic drugs: These highly effective medicines can now be used by a child of any age. Administration is simplified by the use of a holding chamber or a compressor-driven nebulizer.

Theophylline: Long acting preparations release theophylline more slowly and evenly than regular preparations. They require less frequent administration and cause fewer adverse effects.

Cromolyn: This drug has proved to be extremely effective in preventing episodes in many children who have chronic asthma. It causes virtually no adverse effects.

Oral steroids: Short bursts of steroids are now judged a safe and effective home treatment for children with severe episodes of asthma.

Inhaled steroids: These preparations have proved useful for the prevention of asthma episodes in many children who require long-term daily medication.

Parent involvement: Many parents and doctors realize they must work as partners in order to provide the best possible care for children with asthma. Informed parents provide essential information which physicians can use to modify their child's treatment plan.

Each of these advances provides a significant margin of improvement for many children with asthma. Combined, they are truly powerful. Well-informed parents who understand the management of asthma can now make reliable judgments about their children's situation. They can control most episodes without panic according to a plan worked out in advance with their physician. Almost all children with asthma can now lead normal lives, taking part in all sports and social activities.

When I came to Amherst in 1977 to join a group practice, I found that asthma was the most common chronic illness facing my patients. In only a few of these children was the problem controlled to the fullest extent possible. Parents had little understanding of asthma or the functions of the various medications used to treat it.

Over the years I have developed an approach for working with parents based on the following assumptions. Parents can't treat asthma unless they can recognize the early clues and trouble signs that it exhibits and they can't regulate medication dosage unless they know the functions and adverse effects of the drugs used to treat it. To help parents gain control over their children's illness I spend a lot of time trying to describe the workings of asthma to them. I also discuss medications, their desired effects, and their adverse effects. I have written handouts covering these subjects and improvements in asthma care in order to give parents something to refer to, to save time and to reduce the duration and cost of a visit.

Today we care for more than four hundred children with asthma in our pediatric practice. As in the case of every chronic illness, we believe the parents should take on the role of the physician and the physician should serve as their consultant. The parents should observe their child's symptoms and physical state and make management decisions within limits set by their physician consultant.

We expect the parents to be active participants in the care of their child's asthma. We do our best to support them, providing easy access to the office, twenty-four hour availability in case a serious problem occurs, and we encourage them to manage the child's problem at home to the best of their ability. Parents grow in their ability to care for their child with asthma as they learn more about it; during office visits, from our parents' group, from reading, from experience with the child, and from conversations with parents of other children who have asthma.

The parents of all of our patients lead busy lives. Many have full-time jobs. Many have other children. Many are single. Some are full-time students. A number of them live far from the office. It is important for each of them to learn when they can handle a problem themselves and when to come in for help. No parent wants to come in too soon, but if he or she waits too long, it will be more difficult to treat an episode.

At the first visit for an episode of wheezing, we give the parents several handouts. "What is Asthma?" (see p. 39) summarizes the changes that take place in the bronchioles during an asthma episode. Another sheet lists the four signs of asthma trouble. A third sheet, a simple chart to record changes in the child's condition, helps us to relate these changes to medication and to certain triggers. (All of these are described in chapter two.) During this initial visit, parents also receive descriptions of adrenergic drugs and theophylline as well as printed instructions for administration of medication.

During this visit we teach them how to judge the ratio of breathing in (inspiration) to breathing out (expiration). We also point out how to identify sucking in of the chest skin (retraction) and how this lessens with treatment. Finally, we demonstrate how to count the child's breathing rate and discuss the cause and significance of wheezing. In a few minutes of instruction, the parent learns how to judge the severity of each sign. In the future, this parent will be able to detect improvement or worsening after giving medication and will be able to decide whether a visit or call to the doctor is necessary. The parent also acquires the vocabulary needed to communicate clearly with the physician by telephone.

If the child is moderately ill with the first asthma episode, the parent and I stay in contact by phone. We schedule a follow-up visit from one to seven days later. At that time we review the asthma record and answer the parents' questions about medications, asthma, and the process of assessing the severity of the episode. After parents have been guided through their first asthma episode, they develop confidence as they learn from each new experience. Within a few months they begin to say, "Asthma is a nuisance, not a tragedy."

1

Living with Asthma

The parents you are about to meet all have children with asthma. Parents of our patients usually find that they gain skill and confidence by meeting with other mothers and fathers like them, parents who are providing care that is intended to prevent asthma episodes when possible and treat them rapidly when they occur. The parents—whose stories follow—tell, in their own words, of their personal experiences in dealing with children who have asthma.

Casey's mother writes that understanding of her son's asthma "is the best gift anyone has ever given me." Dana Parker captures the physical and emotional trauma of his son's first episode of asthma and tells how his family deals with asthma episodes now. Jeamie Duffy chronicles the first seven years in her son Matthew's life. We learn of the reactions of neighbors and friends and of her own evolution from an asthma-obsessed mother to a parent with appropriate concerns.

Marilyn Sansouci's son Nathan was hospitalized four times in five months but not once in the two years since he started an aggressive treatment program. Harriet Goodwin describes Josh's early symptoms, her dealings with doctors and teachers, and her learning about asthma over a ten-year period. Marjorie Syriac, Heather's mother, learned how to treat asthma during a thirty-six hour hospital stay. Gail Wall, the mother of a teenager, asks for help prior to her first asthma consultation.

Casey

■

CAROLINE TROPP

Casey was approximately fifteen months old when he was diagnosed as having asthma. It started as a cold, then grew much worse. We brought him to a pediatrician who gave him an injection of epinephrine and some medicine by mouth. Because I hadn't known anyone with asthma, I had no idea of the severity of his problem. I didn't know what his illness would entail and how it would affect our future. Casey's doctor told me to give him medicine, which seemed to make him better. Casey took it for a few days and he was fine. A week or two after I stopped the medicine he started wheezing, coughing, and moaning—just like the first time. It was then that I realized that asthma would affect not only Casey, but the whole family.

Every time Casey would have an episode (usually in the middle of the night) we would take him to the emergency room and pray that they could bring his attack under control. Usually we would bring him home. Three times the episode was so severe that he was admitted to the hospital for a few days. If you've ever had a child in the hospital, you know the pain and the helplessness that you feel. When they tell you to go home and your baby is screaming for you to stay, it tears your heart out to leave him there.

Well, this went on for about two years. It seemed that as soon as Casey started to get a cold or the flu, it would bring on an asthma episode. We would give him his medicine and pray. He often ended up in the hospital emergency room. It put a strain on all of us. We didn't understand why our beautiful baby boy had such a severe problem. We felt so helpless. I think you blame yourself for not being able to help your child at his time of need. When friends or relatives would phone, their first question was, "How's Casey's asthma?" I was so frustrated about the whole situation that I remember just crying when he would start wheezing because I knew what would be in store for us. The thing that sticks out most in my mind is that the doctors would say that he would probably grow out of it. Big deal! Was that supposed to help me now?

Casey was almost three years old when we had to switch doctors because of a change in my health insurance. I called to see the new doctor about Casey because I wanted him to become familiar with Casey before he had another episode. I was really surprised when the receptionist said that one of the pediatricians was an asthma specialist. I thought to myself maybe we had found someone who could help my little boy.

When we arrived at the office I was hoping that he could help me, but I kept thinking that maybe he, like the others, would just say, "Casey will probably grow out of his asthma." The pediatrician came into the examining room and introduced himself. He started asking me questions about the medication Casey was taking. Well, Casey wasn't taking any one medication. I had about eight medicines in the house in case of an episode. I couldn't remember half of their names, not to mention what they would do for my child. I felt so dumb because all I knew was that my child had asthma. I knew nothing about the causes of the asthma episodes or about the correct doses or the possible side-effects of Casey's medications.

After the pediatrician reviewed the full story of Casey's asthma with me he examined Casey from head to toe. Then we sent Casey to play in the waiting room while we talked. The doctor started by saying "Casey has moderately severe asthma but we will probably be able to prevent him from staying in the hospital again." We (the doctor and I) would become a team in combating his illness. He prescribed medications and explained them fully. Casey would need to take medication daily. We sat for approximately half an hour and discussed Casey and what I had to know about treating him at home.

I thought, "I have finally found someone who can help us." I had been in the dark for so long but was finally starting to see the light at the end of the tunnel. Why did the other doctors assume that they could treat Casey without involving me? Why couldn't I learn how to help? Why wouldn't they take the time to teach me? All the heartache of Casey's illness could have been minimized years ago.

Do you know, my new doctor didn't mention the fact that Casey might grow out of it? His concern is treating him NOW! Casey is doing exceptionally well. He takes medicine daily and has some backup medicine. I finally feel that everything is under control. He has had a few episodes, but I now know how to treat him successfully at home. After all these years, I feel that I am finally in the driver's seat. My doctor is just a phone call away if I need him. Knowledge and understanding of this illness is the best gift anyone has ever given me.

Ryan

■

DANA PARKER

Just before Thanksgiving in 1981, our son Ryan caught a cold, and developed a very bad cough. As he was only three years old we were concerned about him, and gave him a standard dose of kid's aspirin, cough medicine, and sent him to bed. At 3:00 A.M. he was worse. His eyes were puffy and red, his cough was worse and his breathing was shallow, but these symptoms had no special meaning for us.

We saw the pediatrician later that morning. He decided Ryan had asthma and began a course of treatment that is etched in my memory reminding me of how much we learned, how scared we were, and by contrast, how differently we handle the problem now. After six hours in the treatment room at the doctor's office, where he had received four shots of epinephrine, vomited oral medication five times, and received an hour of intravenous theophylline treatment, our limp and exhausted three-year-old son was admitted to the hospital.

He stayed in the hospital for a couple of days. We shared twenty-four-hour companionship with our son through the ordeal until he came home. Almost immediately we began learning about this thing, asthma. We were asked to learn quickly as much as we could about the problem. Almost overnight we became experts at assessing his condition; by looking at the retraction of the chest skin, carefully observing his in to out ratio, and by counting respirations, and listening to the wheeze. We were told that we had the best tools for noting and reporting small but significant changes in Ryan's condition both in a measurable clinical way, and also in that indeterminable way that parents look at their children. We can tell the quality of how the kid feels by the color in his face, the way he speaks and the "droop" of his eyes.

We learned from each of the five asthma episodes that Ryan had over the next four months. Our whole family read the book, *Teaching Myself About Asthma,* and the twenty or so handouts that our doctor demanded that we learn cold. The short course we participated in with other parents of kids with asthma was a big help in tying things together. This education works, for in spite of the subsequent episodes, Ryan has not been back to the hospital.

The way that we have come to treat the problem at our house has developed, quite quickly, from panic and fear into a pretty manageable ritual. Certainly after that first trip to the hospital, we were bound and determined to do better next time. The hospital was the last place I wanted to be with Ryan, unless we had no choice. We were told quite to our amazement that kids don't often require hospitalization, and that indeed, Ryan had had a real bad episode. He is a kid who gets into trouble quickly, and we have to move just as quickly to help. It is clear that the treatment team consists of the three doctors, my wife and myself, Ryan, and our other sons. The clinical assessment of the in to out ratio, retractions, rate of respiration, and wheezing has become something that we do out of habit, sometimes several times a day, and many times a day during an asthma episode. We now know what Ryan looks like before he's going to have an asthma episode. He knows how he feels when it's coming on. Although he is a couple months short of four years, he can tell you what happens to his bronchial tubes during an episode because his brother reads the asthma book to him a lot. When he has an episode, Ryan gets out his big graduated pitcher for drinks because he knows he needs a lot of liquids to get better. And medication.

You know, Ryan can be stubborn. During his first episode we battled over taking theophylline beads. I forced him to swallow them. He vomited them after a short time. I put him in the high chair with the sole intention of getting that medicine into him. We stayed in the kitchen for most of the day and he would not take it. I panicked due to my concern that he might have to go back into the hospital. Finally, out of desperation I called the doctor. He suggested we try giving Ryan liquid theophylline. It worked! Now all is fine except that we have to give medicine every six hours.

Our view is that we prefer to have Ryan at home, and not at the hospital, or even at the doctor's office if we can help it. What has developed over the last six months is absolutely terrific. We have great confidence in our three pediatricians, and they have confidence in us. We often call during an episode to discuss symptoms, medication dose, adverse effects, and ultimately to decide whether we can handle the situation at home. As we learn, we have become more able to help Ryan directly and we feel much more confident about trusting our own judgment. Because we now share a common medical language with our pediatricians, consultation can take place over the phone. This has helped us move from feeling like helpless victims of this illness, to being an active part of the "getting better" process. We are surprised at how many trips to the office we have avoided, and how reassuring it is for Ryan to be in his own house, his own bed, hearing the familiar sounds of home.

We also have become more aware of the things that trigger Ryan's asthma. When Ryan has a cold, we start giving him medicines. When it's below 32 degrees outside, he wears a mask, and is only out for brief periods of time. On his own, Ryan avoids dusty and "bad air" situations. He doesn't like asthma problems either.

We have struggled with asthma as a family, but I think that we are winning. Trying to work, stay normal, pay attention to the other children, sleep at night, avoid arguing due to over-tiredness, control the anger coming from old impressions of asthma that remain . . . this is hard work. The results, however, have been gratifying. We are delighted that we can call the office and speak with a doctor who knows us well and trusts our judgment.

You should also know that Ryan, in spite of his asthma, and in spite of how quickly he gets into trouble, is a tough, active, athletic little kid. He climbs anything with a foothold, runs like the wind, and rarely tires.

I firmly believe that while asthma is scary and quite serious, it is quite manageable. We could have remained victims of our fear, but we did not. We hope that Ryan's body will begin to grow as predicted and that his windpipes will enlarge significantly, and therefore relieve some of the problem. This may happen between the ages of four and six. If his asthma problem continues, we know how to help him, and he is getting better at knowing how to help himself.

We don't know everything about asthma, but we know a lot about our son's asthma. We all work hard at it, and the fear is gone from the situation. We feel pretty good about how we handle it, and it makes Ryan feel better when we can show him that confidence.

Matthew

■

JEAMIE DUFFY

Matthew's story really begins before his birth. My husband and I both have asthma and we were prepared for an allergic child. I have outgrown my asthma; my husband, however, would still be called moderately severe. My father, a physician, warned us when we were first married to carefully consider the decision to have children because of our allergic histories. Luckily, we followed our desire to have at least one child.

Because we were prepared, Matthew's bedroom was never cluttered with stuffed animals, toys or knick-knacks. There were never any animals to remove from our home. His bedroom contained a crib, a dresser and a lamp. To this day it remains the same.

Matthew's first sign of trouble came when he was about five months old. He was lying on the floor, munching on a cracker when suddenly I heard that very familiar wheeze. I have to emphasize that we were ready for this. I knew what wheezing sounded like. I knew that he would not stop breathing. I also knew that he needed to be treated. In this sense, we were lucky. I can imagine the frightening feeling of seeing and hearing your infant have trouble breathing and not knowing exactly what was happening or what to do.

The first episode was mild. Liquid theophylline for a few days was all that he needed. The biggest problem was convincing the doctor that he had asthma. He had trouble believing that Matthew's trouble would start so early or that the parents could identify the problem themselves. By the time he was a year old, Matt had undergone two more mild episodes and we had moved to Amherst, Massachusetts. By that time, he was on a maintenance dose of theophylline and was becoming quite sensitive to allergies. He was underweight and had "the look." He often had dark circles under his eyes, got eczema from certain foods and had a constant stuffy nose.

By age two, Matthew's asthma was getting worse, as was my husband's. That spring was bad! Matthew spent Mother's Day at the hospital with a full-fledged flare and I was beginning to get upset. My husband Joe would go to the emergency room one evening and Matthew would follow a few days later. I once remarked to my mother that I was hearing stereo wheezing throughout the house.

At this time, I was beginning to let Matthew's asthma become the focal point in my life. This obsession lasted for about two and a half years. In retrospect, it was not good for anyone. My obsession took the form of over-protection and his illness was constantly on my mind. I was afraid to let him near a child with a cough for fear he'd catch cold. I was afraid to let him near an animal for fear it would trigger his wheezing.

I became compulsive about keeping the house clean. I dusted and vacuumed every day to maintain the perfect dust-free environment. This parental effort can be very important, but I went overboard. I still try to keep a clean house, but now I clean every other day or so. I clean now because I want to have a dust-free home, not because I'm driven to keep a dust-free home.

I was also beginning to feel very sorry for myself. I talked about Matthew's problem to anyone that would listen. Every asthma episode was reported in detail, to friends, family, and even strangers. I needed to talk about his problem to "get it off my chest." Yes, his asthma was bad, but I made it appear worse than it was as I talked about it with friends. Looking back, I think I wanted sympathy. After an attack, I was very tired and wanted someone to take care of me for a while. Trying to be a Super Mom is exhausting!

Joe and I never disagreed about Matthew's health; we reacted to it differently. He never went to the extremes that I did. One of the reasons I think this was so is because he had a full-time profession and I didn't. He could walk away in the morning to an apparently exciting job, and away from Matt's health. I, on the other hand, was surrounded by Matthew's illness. He was not in school so I had nothing to divert my attention. Each cough meant another flare, more epinephrine, more nights awake; the circle never stopped.

This was also the time when we began to discuss the size of our family. We had always said that we wanted two kids, but now we were questioning whether we actually wanted another. We couldn't see having another child with asthma; it was expensive, it was tiring, and it was emotionally draining. We decided against another child. Rather, we put off thinking about it for a while. The subject would come up in discussion every six months or so, but always with the same result—let's wait.

When Matthew was three years old, he needed his first dose of steroids. I don't think I will ever forget that day. It was the 4th of July weekend—we were playing "hide and seek" and I could find Matthew easily by listening for his wheeze and cough. After a few shots of epinephrine, it was obvious that he needed something more; he began his first course of prednisone. To me, that meant he had reached another level of his illness—a more serious level. Prior to this, shots of epinephrine and theophylline capsules would break an attack.

Despite all of this, Matthew was growing up to be a happy, normal child. He took his illness in stride. As a matter of fact, he never thought of himself as being ill. He thought that all kids took medicine every day. He thought everyone's eyes itched when they were near animals. He thought everyone needed shots to help them breathe. His dad did all these things—why not everyone?

Joe and I strongly believed that if we paid too much attention to Matt's chronic illness he would grow up with an emotional illness too. We were straightforward about his restrictions (food, animals, etc.), but we spoke of these in the same tone that we warned him about playing with matches. He never saw himself as being different. We always let him determine how much physical activity he could handle. We never stopped him from playing ball, running or other vigorous activities. There were times when we wanted to. But we felt that if we interfered, he and his friends would think of him as being different. Then he would always have a crutch when things did not go his way: "I'm wheezy and I can't go to bed," "I have asthma, therefore I need and deserve special attention."

I especially wanted to stop him once when a group of children were playing tag in our front yard. One child was "it" and the rest ran around trying not to get caught. Matthew was having trouble with his asthma, still playing, but never running away. He moved *in place,* but he never moved from that one spot. None of the children realized what he was doing, but I watched from the front window. Our child refused to be different, our child refused to be sick. Matthew was "one of the kids." I wanted to stop that game and substitute a quiet one, but I didn't. It was important for Matthew to learn to make judgments and set his own limits.

Joe and I are proud of the fact that Matthew does not feel sorry for himself or think of himself as being different. It is hard not to buy some special toy for him when he is sick; it is hard not to wait on him hand and foot when he is having an episode. We want to do special things for him, but when a child has a chronic illness you would always be doing that special thing. Then you're in trouble. I remember when Matthew was three-and-a-half, he had an especially bad episode that lasted days, with numerous trips to the doctor and a lot of shots. This was when Matthew first asked for a Big Wheel. During the episode, I wanted to go out and buy the Big Wheel and tell him that he was so good about the shots that we bought him the bike. Instead, we waited for about three weeks and then gave it to him, saying that we were proud of him and that he was a good boy. He knew he was getting rewarded for being good, not for being sick.

The regimen of medication became difficult at this time. He now took prednisone frequently and this presented a problem. Prednisone came only in pill form then and Matthew did not swallow pills. This meant crushing the pill and mixing it with applesauce. A crushed prednisone pill tastes worse than a crushed aspirin—I know because I tried it. We also had to wake him up at night to give him his theophylline, but Matthew never cried or complained.

Another problem caused by the medication was the behavior changes that they provoked. Theophylline, for example, can cause nervousness and jumpiness. Prednisone can cause mood swings, both high and low. Matthew gets exuberant on the prednisone; we recognized that right away. Finally, metaproterenol tablets cause his hands to shake. These side effects created a problem with discipline. If Matthew acted up, being fresh or belligerent, we felt (at times) that it was because of the medication. But we also felt that the behavior had to be stopped. If he got away with this behavior while on medication, he would surely try it again while off of it. It is difficult to punish your child for something he might not have control over—but you know you must.

Other people's reactions to Matthew were quite varied. A few examples can best show this. When Matthew was about three-and-a-half, we went to the grocery store soon after an episode. Though the wheezing had stopped, he was still coughing. Matthew's cough is loud and deep; once he broke a few blood vessels in his face from coughing so hard. While we were shopping, he started to cough. A woman passed me in the aisle, listened to Matthew, and shook her head. We passed her again a few aisles later and Matthew was still coughing. The woman stopped me and asked me how I had the nerve to take such a sick child outside. At first I wanted to explain, then I wanted to yell at her that it was none of her business. I did neither. She walked away shaking her head, probably thinking I was an incompetent mother. I left the store angry!

Fortunately, for every embarrassing situation, there are many more like the following. Our next door neighbors have a boy just Matthew's age and they became best friends. They have a cat, which means that Matthew can never go inside their house to play. That is not a problem in the spring or summer, but winter is hard. After Matthew had to miss Ray's birthday party because of the cat, they gave the cat away. Of course, we never asked or expected them to do so. They realized on their own how hard it was on Matthew. I hope I never forget the feeling I got when Ray's mother told me why they gave the cat away. She said that Matthew and Ray's friendship was more important and would last longer than the cat.

In the spring, when Matthew was about four years old, he had a very bad time. It seemed that we were at the doctor's office every day and sometimes twice a day. Luckily, by this time he had learned to swallow pills and to use an inhaler, which made medicating easier. His asthma seemed to be getting worse, and I was very down. Part of my depression, I'm sure, came from lack of sleep, but I also saw this illness as an ongoing thing that was beginning to overwhelm me. Each episode was sure to subside, but it was also sure that he would have another soon. I talked about it with my dad, a pediatrician. He told us that very soon Matthew would outgrow his problem, or at least get much better. For the next ten months, Matthew had very little trouble. He was still taking daily medication, but every cold no longer triggered an attack. We were thrilled. We were even ready to consider having another child. I was convinced that Matthew was outgrowing his asthma and would soon be fine. We even spoke to the doctor about tapering him off his daily medications.

This interlude did not last. The next spring came along and Matthew was even worse. Again, there were multiple episodes and trips to the doctor. I felt crushed. I had convinced myself that Matthew was better. Now, in addition to coping with an attack, I had to face the fact that he had not outgrown the problem. It was a double whammy that spring. It took a long time for me to get out of that depression. Probably the best thing I did was to get a part-time job when he started kindergarten.

With a new job, I had more to think about than a clean house, Matthew's cough, and juggling medicines. My work in the morning, while he was in school, gave me an outlet for my energy and a new focus for my thought. My obsession with Matthew's health began to subside. It was not an immediate, but a gradual lessening of my emotional involvement. Over a period of months I began to accept the fact that Matthew had a chronic illness, but not a debilitating one. Yes, he was limited in certain ways, but overall he was able to live a normal life and so should I. Of course, Joe and I were still concerned when he had an episode, but we also knew that he would come out of it and go right back to being an active, happy boy. He still took a lot of medication, but now it was much easier. We had worked out a comfortable schedule for medication. He had to take a theophylline capsule at 4:00 P.M. every day. The neighbors used to say they could set their clocks by the time I got on my bike with pill and water, trying to find Matthew who was playing outside. We no longer had to wake him during the night to give medication—he got a larger dose before bed—and we all slept better.

The doctors we take Matthew to believe that parents who know what is happening are the best diagnosticians for their child. Thanks to them, we know how medications work, what their side effects are and how to judge the severity of an attack. We know how to determine if he is getting worse and what action to take. Put simply, we know what to do. I can honestly say that I know when Matthew is getting bad even before the actual signs appear. People (and doctors) ask what it is that tells me this. I cannot put it into words. It's a combination of the way he acts and the way he looks. If we took him to the doctor when I sensed that he was getting bad, probably the doctor would not hear a lot of wheezing or see outward signs. Luckily, our doctors trust us as parents and listen to us. I feel Matthew has been kept healthier because of this.

Matthew was hospitalized again at age five. Although the intravenous infusion and blood tests hurt Matthew, he did not get upset and I did not get depressed. Whenever Matthew has to undergo an uncomfortable procedure like a blood test he never cries or complains. I believe he senses that this is what he needs to get better. I am not the religious type, but I do believe God gives children with chronic illnesses a little extra something. That something might take the form of patience or acceptance.

Since then, Matthew has been scratch tested for allergies (we were not surprised when he showed up positive) and begun allergy shots. We have seen some improvement since then. His asthma is better controlled with medication and his episodes are less frequent.

Matthew is seven years old now. He had to be hospitalized again recently but bounced back quickly. The afternoon of his discharge, he was outside riding his bike. Joe and I still have our moments of being down, and there are times when I want to start feeling very sorry for myself and Matthew; but when those feelings begin I look at our family as a whole and have to be happy. This afternoon Matthew is out in the front yard with ten neighbors playing baseball. He is a happy child—full of fun and energy. He can do all those "normal" things. If he starts to wheeze while playing, he just calls "time out," comes in to use his inhaler, and runs back out again.

Nathan

■

MARILYN SANSOUCI

Our fourth son, Nathan, was born in April 1981. He weighed eight pounds, ten ounces and was a very handsome little fellow. We were very pleased with him. He was healthy and fine until one day in November when he caught a cold. We treated it with aspirin and a decongestant. This didn't seem to help him at all. By the third day he became worse. He began to cough quite frequently and he was breathing rapidly. By the time evening came, our baby was struggling to breathe. We immediately called an ambulance which took us to the hospital. He was put in an oxygen tent for several days. After taking chest x-rays, the doctor said that our son had pneumonia. He gave him an antibiotic and after a week's stay in the hospital, Nathan was sent home. He did fine for three weeks but when he caught another cold it turned into a nightmare.

Late one night I awoke from a sound sleep with a feeling that I should look in on the baby. I check on all the boys every night (a mother's routine) before I go to bed, but this time it was different. When I went into Nathan's room I heard him wheezing and coughing and gasping for air. I ran and woke my husband. We rushed our baby to the hospital and on the way total fear gripped me. I feared that this time we were going to lose our son. By the time we got to the hospital, Nathan's lips began to turn blue from lack of oxygen. He was put into an oxygen tent again, and all we could do was pray to God that our baby would be all right. I believe it was a miracle, an answer to prayer, that Nathan did survive. They took more chest x-rays and did a test for cystic fibrosis, which were negative, and we were very thankful for that.

I remember feeling distressed and wondering how long this would continue before we would find out what was causing our little boy to get so sick so often. When I was to bring Nathan home from the hospital approximately one week later, I called his doctor to ask if he had made a diagnosis yet. He told me there was still no diagnosis and encouraged me just to be happy he was better. Well, by this time I had had my fill of finding out nothing concerning my baby. Certainly we were happy that he was better, but for how long? We knew something was terribly wrong but we just didn't know what. We decided it was time to change doctors. At this time we were referred to another pediatrician by a friend. The first time we visited this new doctor and I told him of Nathan's trauma, he diagnosed him as having asthma and began treatment with theophylline three times a day. Despite this treatment, Nathan was still hospitalized for asthma twice more before his first birthday.

In March of 1982 we joined a health maintenance organization. The next time Nathan had an asthma episode, he was examined by our new family doctor, who then phoned for a pediatric consultation. After he got off the phone he ordered three shots for Nathan. I believe the shots were epinephrine twice, followed by a long-acting epinephrine preparation. Nathan responded and was able to go home within an hour. He continued treatment with theophylline capsules and prednisone three times a day for a short period of time. This was the first time that he had an asthma episode and was not admitted to the hospital. We were so thrilled to be able to take our baby home the same night. It was beautiful not to have to go home to an empty crib. This was the beginning of learning about our son's asthma.

Nathan was fine for about a month and then he had another episode. This time the pediatrician increased the theophylline dose but Nathan couldn't tolerate the full amount. He got hyperactive and wouldn't sleep at night. He did calm down after it was reduced. The consulting pediatrician prescribed metaproterenol followed by cromolyn, both delivered by a compressor-driven nebulizer three times a day. This amounts to a regular program of treatment and prevention at the same time.

Not long ago my family doctor recommended that my husband and I attend the Parents' Asthma Group that was held in Amherst. We attended two two-hour sessions and are very glad we did. We learned a lot about asthma and how to detect episodes early and how to monitor these episodes. We also learned about various medicines used to treat asthma, their good effects and also their undesirable effects. It was good to share experiences with other parents: to hear what they were going through and how it affected them. It helps to know that we are not the only parents going through these problems.

In the beginning of Nathan's sickness, we feared for his life. At the Parents' Asthma Group we learned that it was rare for a child to die of asthma. Only one of every 25,000 children with asthma die of it each year. If parents have adequate knowledge and see that their children get proper treatment, this tiny number will become smaller still.

Nathan is now three years old and doing much better. In the two years he has been on this new treatment plan, he hasn't been admitted to the hospital once. He takes theophylline capsules twice a day except when he begins a cold, then I'll add another capsule at night. He takes metaproterenol and cromolyn by nebulizer three times a day. Since we've learned more about how to deal with Nathan's condition and he's on this medication, he has gone as long as three months without an episode. Before he was having them at least once a month. What an improvement!

Josh

■

HARRIET GOODWIN

"How long has this baby been wheezing?" asked the pediatrician in Peterborough, New Hampshire. We had all been praying for his arrival as the few general practitioners were so overworked. He didn't ask this question politely. There was a nasty, guilt-producing edge to the question. Like, "Lady, how long have you been so dumb?" In truth, I had brought eighteen-month old Josh in because he had had this odd, sharp cough all morning. There didn't seem to be any cold symptoms. I was torn between ignoring it and taking him in, thereby running the risk of being laughed at as an over-anxious mother.

"What's wheezing?" I asked. And that was how I learned that my second and until now perfectly normal, (well, almost) healthy baby had *asthma.* What a curse! Everyone knew asthma was a psychosomatic disease caused, of course, by mother! Oh God, Sigmund Freud has my number. This is it. I thought I had been doing such a good job of faking parenting.

Then came the shot of epinephrine. Then the twenty-minute wait in the waiting room while Josh turned ghastly pale white. Then the slightly congratulatory welcome back to the second shot—well good, epinephrine will work on him. And then the prescription for a combination medicine (asthma syrup), to be administered every few hours for the next few days and then, after that, as needed. There was probably a follow-up visit. It's hard to remember. Josh is almost twelve. He was born in 1970. So this story starts about nine and a half years back.

When Josh was three years old we determined that he was allergic to peanuts. We moved shortly after and our new pediatrician advised us to see an allergist to define this problem and get advice on the care of Josh's frequent wheezing. The allergist said that Josh was allergic to peanuts and prescribed an epinephrine kit.

The years between Josh at age three, with "occasional" asthma, and Josh at seven, when our "awakening" to the true nature of his condition occurred, are something of a blur to me. I don't remember using the asthma syrup very often.

When Josh went to kindergarten at age five, the teacher called and told me that he seemed more comfortable with the "fours" and seemed to belong there. That was fine with me, as I could tell that he was nowhere near being ready to deal with even the pre-reading. He was quite small for his age as well. His constant runny nose as well as his small, skinny size, made him seem a bit sickly, I guess.

Josh's first grade teacher said he often appeared tired and would nap under her desk during the afternoon. The next year his second grade teacher recommended a full evaluation of Josh's social, psychological and educational status. The school psychiatric consultant diagnosed Josh as being chronically depressed.

On our first visit to the psychiatrist he commented that Josh seemed very unwell. We agreed and said that perhaps April was a poor month for Josh allergy-wise. That night, Josh had his first really severe asthma flare in a long time. We brought him to the office to see the new pediatrician who had recently taken over the practice. In between the first shot of epinephrine and the second one, he grilled us. What were we doing for this child's wheezing? Again I felt that pang of guilt that I had experienced in Peterborough.

The doctor seemed astounded and appalled when I told him that I gave Josh medication only if I heard him wheeze. "You've got to continue medication for at least two days after wheezing stops," he said. Patiently, he explained that he was reluctant to prescribe medicine unless necessary, but most people don't treat an episode long enough.

My little boy had asthma. It was as if I had never heard the words before. Deep shock set in. I had a very close friend who suffered terribly from asthma. This friend used to tell me that

Josh was wheezing. I would bring Josh to swim at his lake cottage and he would say, "Harriet, Josh is wheezing." "Oh, it's nothing," I would say. At this time Josh was four or five years old. Not my Josh, he didn't have asthma. Not like that. When my friend dropped over, saw Josh, he said warningly, "He's wheeeeeezing." Why hadn't I taken it more seriously? I will never know. Perhaps just ignorance. I do know that it wasn't just Josh who had to be treated. We, Josh's father, Mike, and I, now had to be educated right along with Josh.

The first revelation was about the asthma syrup. Combination medicines are no longer recommended by the experts, said Josh's doctor. They contain unnecessary ingredients which can lead to bad side effects. So it was out with the combo and in with the theophylline. We had one phyllin, this phyllin and that phyllin. At last, we settled on a long-acting theophylline tablet and taught Josh to master the fine art of pill-swallowing. What a breakthrough that was! Liberation from pouring liquids into those plastic measuring-spoons, and dribbling it down the poor child's throat. All the while, the pediatrician provided support for Mike and me as we learned about asthma. Josh was always quite calm about all these new medical developments as one episode followed another that April. As I remember it, we went to the office for epinephrine shots at least four times or more in ten days.

When our pediatrician decided to run a class for parents of children with asthma, our names were high up on the list of candidates for this series of meetings. Even as he worked on evaluating Josh's medication, adding, changing, deleting, improving, listening to those lungs and listening again, our worst fears were alleviated by these wonderful classes. After hearing what some of the other parents had been through and were going through, we realized that Josh was not as badly off as we had thought. I can't describe what a relief it was to finally, once and for all, understand that Josh would not die in the ten minute interval between our house and the doctor's office, no matter how bad he sounded.

We learned about all of the different kinds of asthma medicines, how they work, and why they are chosen for use. We learned that lung damage from asthma is rare indeed. We began to face the probability that Josh would take medicine for years, and that he might not ever "outgrow" it, although no one could predict anything and I still, to this day, hope that he will. We learned how to judge the severity of a flare by looking at the retractions at his neck. We were taught how to use the stethoscope and instructed in its use as a diagnostic tool at home. And then came the endless (or so it seemed) months of keeping a record, listening three times a day, writing down in a sort of code a day-by-day description of his condition.

I began to feel that I was partly the doctor. There were many consultations (by phone and in the office) during this initial period of treatment which stretched over a year or more. At last we arrived at an effective combination of long-acting theophylline, metaproterenol and anti-histamine. During this time, our pediatrician seemed to be constantly attending seminars on this stubborn disease, and trying new ideas. He liberalized his attitude toward the inhaler, and taught us to use it right along with the other medications. I think that was the final refinement, and it serves us in good stead. Our rule is that Josh may use the inhaler three times a day, but after that the doctor wants to hear about it and, most likely, to see him. This has almost never occurred.

It came as a big surprise to me when, last year, I had to be reminded that it was time to bring Josh in for a checkup. He had gone to the doctor's so often in the past that it never occurred to me that three months might slip by without a visit.

Josh underwent another series of allergy tests, but no strategic information turned up. He had his serum theophylline level checked several times. We increased his dose to 400 mg twice a day, which I thought was a lot, but it seemed to be just right for treating our seventy-pound boy.

This May, Josh had his first bad episode in over a year. I attribute much of this good track record to intelligent and discriminate use of theophylline and the inhaler. One of the most important things I remember learning from the Parents' Asthma Group is how one episode leaves the lungs in a susceptible condition for some forty-eight hours after the symptoms have gone. This placed our treatment approach in context for me and helped me to accept it.

I finally rebelled against keeping records after Josh had been quite well for a long time. I put away my stethoscope several years ago (although it is always there if I need it). I have learned to get all the lung information I need by pressing my ear right up to a bare chest.

Josh is now almost completely in control of his own medication. Once in a while there are complications. Just two days ago, he forgot he had taken his evening medicine and took it again. He was up a good part of the night vomiting and enduring stomach pain. Josh leaves me a note when it is time to refill the prescription. He had dropped his three o'clock metaproterenol and allergy pill for several months over the summer. Just yesterday, I saw a big note that he left for himself on the kitchen counter near his pills:

JOSH TAKE YOUR THREE O'CLOCK PILLS

Josh is now in the fifth grade, reading on an early sixth-grade level. He repeated a year, and thanks to the superb special education teachers and the proper medication routine, he is now back in a regular classroom. He is a happy and highly motivated boy. His depression in the second grade was probably related to his inadequately treated asthma. At last I am an educated parent with an educated child who knows about his asthma. I wouldn't have it any other way.

Heather

■

MARJORIE SYRIAC

Heather was about five months old when she got sick. She had been really fussy all day long. I thought maybe she had an earache so I called the doctor's office and the nurse said to bring her in. It is a twenty mile drive and we got there at 8:00 P.M. I also had to bring Heather's two older brothers with me because their dad was working. When we got to the office Heather was worse than she had been all day. Her temperature was up and she seemed to be having trouble breathing.

Heather's pediatrician saw us right away and checked her over. He told me that she did have an ear infection, but the main problem was that she was having an asthma episode. He showed me that Heather was sucking in the skin below her breast bone and in between her ribs. It was taking her a lot longer to breathe out than to breathe in and she was breathing forty-two times a minute. She was not wheezing at all. The thought of asthma scared me. I had never had to deal with anything like that before.

The doctor took us into the treatment room and gave Heather some liquid theophylline. She vomited a few minutes later. Then he said he was going to treat her with metaproterenol mist. He set up the machine and explained how to measure the medicine. Then he held Heather in his arms and put a mask up to her face and turned on the machine. The mist was supposed to open up the air passages and make it easier for her to breathe. After about two minutes the doctor asked me to take over. Heather didn't like it at all. She cried and tried to push the mask away from her face. The doctor said the crying would help because she was breathing deeper and would pull more medicine into her lungs. This went on for about ten minutes. Then he shut off the machine and checked Heather's breathing again. He said she had improved some, but not enough for me to bring her home since I had no idea how to deal with the medications or how to decide whether she was getting better or worse. She would have to be admitted to the hospital. The nursing staff would get us through this episode and teach me how to care for Heather at home.

The pediatrician called Guy (Heather's father) and repeated what he had told me. Then he called the hospital to tell them that we were coming in. By the time we got to the hospital it was almost midnight. I knew I couldn't stay overnight because I had the two other children with me. So I stayed until she fell asleep and then went home.

The next morning I got a sitter for the kids and Guy and I went to the hospital. We tried to feed Heather but she wanted nothing to do with it. We worked with the nurses and respiratory therapists as they gave her medicines and treatments. At noon I left for home to take a shower and to get enough clothes for the night. Then I went back to the hospital and let Guy go home to be with the other kids. It was one of the longest nights I've ever had. It seemed that every time I got Heather to sleep someone would come in and wake her up for a treatment or to check her breathing. They would explain what they were doing but I was too tired to learn about asthma that night.

In the morning the doctor came in and told me that Heather could go home if I felt ready to handle her by myself. I had learned the four signs of asthma trouble so I could check Heather's progress. I said I would have no problem with the medicines if a nurse would sit down with me to help me get the medicine routines in writing. That way when my alarm clock goes off at 2:00 A.M. I could just look at the paper to see what medication she was supposed to get.

We left the hospital at noon, just thirty-six hours after we had arrived. On the way home I stopped at the doctor's office to pick up the compressor-driven nebulizer to make the meta-proterenol mist. Now I knew how to use it. The first few days were hard. Heather was taking metaproterenol mist every four hours, liquid theophylline every six hours, and prednisone several times a day. She also took an antibiotic three times a day for her ear infection. Many times I would wake up at night when the alarm went off and just sit there on the bed trying to figure out what I was supposed to do; but it did get easier as time went on.

Two days after we got out of the hospital we went back to the office for a check-up. Heather was acting fine except she was sleeping more than usual—catching up, I guess. The doctor said she looked good to him and told me to stop giving predni-sone. We changed over to long acting theophylline (every twelve hours instead of every six) and starting reducing her mist treat-ments. We agreed to get rid of one medicine at a time step by step until she didn't need any. And that is what happened.

Heather did really well without medicine for about three weeks. We had no problem at all. However one night she fell asleep early. I just let her sleep on the couch for a while and then moved her to her crib. As I carried her I noticed that she was having trouble breathing. I watched her for a while and noted that her ribs were showing as she took each breath.

I knew she was having another asthma episode. I called the office to ask if I should bring Heather in. The doctor said that I could handle the problem if I used the same schedule we had worked out when she came home from the hospital. But if I felt that I couldn't handle things I should bring her to the office. I sat back for a minute and thought about it. Before I had a chance to say anything he said, "I know you can do it. I am on duty all night. If anything comes up, just call me." That made me feel a lot better, and we got through that episode without difficulty.

For about three months Heather continued to have asthma episodes. I took care of them myself, using the plan I had worked out with the doctor. Each time it happened it got a little bit easier, but it still took a lot out of everyone. It got to the point where I was waking up in the middle of the night, trying to remember if she was supposed to have any medicines.

When Heather was sixteen months old the doctor mentioned that we might be able to prevent some of her asthma episodes by using a medicine called cromolyn along with the metaproterenol in her mist machine. That meant she would have to use the machine three or four times a day, every day. It would be a lot of work. After discussing it with Guy I decided to try the cromolyn. For the next six months Heather took cromolyn and metaproterenol three or four times a day. She didn't have a single asthma episode. Then we decided to stop the treatments to see how she would do. Well, Heather had only one flare in the fifteen months since then. I suppose she'll have another episode sometime but we are now ready to handle it.

Russ
■
GAIL WALL

It was on Russell's sixth birthday when I knew he had a breathing problem that was not going to go away. We had the family and other guests at the house to celebrate his birthday. It was March, cold and windy. He came into the house, sat on my lap and said, "I can't breathe again." I held him, talked to him and stroked his cheek until he said, "I'm OK now."

When Russ had a cold our family doctor treated him with antibiotics. After his death, we started going to a pediatrician. I told the new doctor Russell's history as best as I could. From then on Russ's colds were treated with a shot of epinephrine as well as antibiotics.

Russell joined a hockey league when he was ten years old. It was evident at this point that sitting on Mom's lap and being treated with antibiotics and a shot of epinephrine was not going to help him breathe well enough to play hockey. But he stuck it out. Sometimes he had to come off the ice after a few minutes.

We moved to a new town and went to another pediatrician. Believe it or not, he was the first doctor to use the word asthma! He prescribed theophylline for the episodes. Russell had stomach upsets and could not sleep when he took this medicine. However, I felt that we were making progress.

This pediatrician left his practice when Russell was fourteen. Since then Russ and I have coped as best we could. His only treatment has been emergency room visits. When I telephone the pediatrician's office I may reach three different pediatricians in a twelve-hour period. Each one gives different instructions.

Now Russ is eighteen years old. In April and in June his asthma flared up. We made three trips to the emergency room with each episode and things were worse than ever. Russ was very sick from this last attack. He had a violent headache and severe vomiting from too much theophylline. One doctor said stop the theophylline, one said continue it, and the third said switch to terbutaline. At this point I said, "————— I've had it! There is a doctor out there who knows how to deal with this and I'm going to find him!" I did. I called for an appointment and now I am trying to put my son's asthma history down on paper.

Russ is intelligent, talented (he will be an architect), and athletic. Yes, he is good at soccer, hockey and baseball and he would be an excellent athlete if we could master his asthma.

And he is dead set against drugs. Theophylline is a drug. Yesterday Russ had a severe headache. I called and talked to one doctor who told me to continue the theophylline, add a strong pain killer for the headache, and to come in. We saw another doctor. He said he wasn't sure what to do. Maybe Russ should start taking cromolyn. Russ said, "I'm sick of filling my body with this ————. I can't eat. I can't sleep. I can't work. I don't want a pain killer and a new medication. I want to reach my potential. And these drugs I'm filling my body with aren't helping. I want my body clean."

We went home and he took two puffs of his inhaler. A few hours later, more inhaler. He was up coughing all night. At 6:00 A.M. after two puffs of the inhaler I took him to work. He is a dishwasher at Howard Johnson's. He got out of the car and said, "Oh, God. I'll call you when I'm through with work." He took a deep breath. Another day to cope.

Russ is a muscular, six foot two inch young man. He is too big to sit on my lap.

Help.

2

Basic Facts

We believe that you can keep your child out of the hospital and the emergency room if you learn some basic facts about asthma and the medications used to treat it. This chapter provides these facts as well as tools to help you judge what is going on during an asthma episode. We teach the four signs of asthma trouble to parents the first time they bring a child to the office with an asthma problem. At the same visit they learn how to keep an asthma record so that they can follow the child's progress during each episode.

This is the essential information that you will need to help you judge what is going on during an asthma episode. Once you know the four signs of asthma trouble and have learned how to keep an asthma record, you will have a solid foundation for working out a home treatment plan with your doctor.

How Do the Lungs Work?

You must know what happens during the normal process of breathing in order to understand what happens during an asthma episode. Breathing provides a continuous supply of oxygen to the body. This oxygen is needed to release energy from the food that we eat and to enable the body cells to do the many jobs that keep us alive. Twenty-one percent of the air that enters our lungs is oxygen.

The illustrations on page 36, 38, 39, 40, 41, 42, and 43 as well as substantial portions of the section on Early Clues, page 53, were adapted from Thomas L. Creer, *Living with Asthma: Part 1. Manual for Teaching Parents the Self-Management of Childhood Asthma.* NIH Publication No. 86–2364; National Heart, Lung, and Blood Institute; Bethesda, Md.; 1986.

Normal Lungs

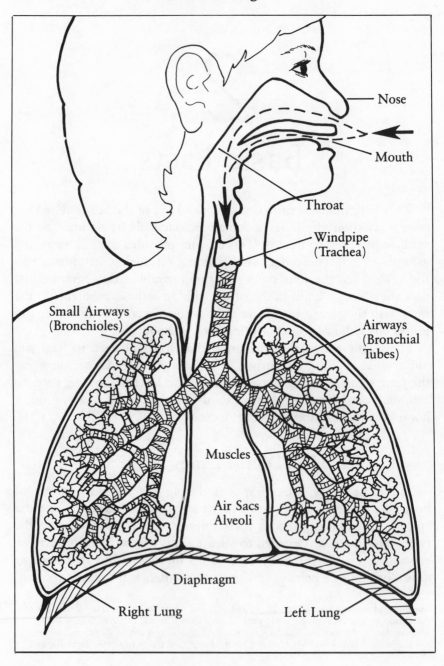

It is absorbed into the blood stream deep inside our lungs. The blood carries oxygen to the billions of cells in the body. As the body cells function, they use up oxygen and produce the gas carbon dioxide, which is exhaled.

ANATOMY OF THE RESPIRATORY SYSTEM

As you breathe in, air flows through the nose or mouth, down the throat (pharynx), through the voice box (larynx), and continues down the windpipe (trachea). The air then reaches the right and left bronchial tubes (bronchi). Bronchial tubes that contain cartilage reinforcement are known as the "large airways" or bronchi. They branch into smaller and smaller passageways called the "small airways" or "bronchioles." The air continues into the bronchioles through ten to twenty-five branches before reaching the three hundred million air sacs (alveoli) where air exchange takes place.

Oxygen leaves the air sacs and enters the tiny, thin blood vessels (capillaries) that surround them (see p. 38). The blood carries oxygen to the body's tissues, including the brain and the heart. At the same time, carbon dioxide leaves the capillaries and enters the air sacs. The carbon dioxide is a waste product of chemical reactions in the body. After entering the air sacs, it is eliminated when a person breathes out.

THE MUSCLES OF BREATHING

The main breathing muscle is the diaphragm (see p. 39). It is the large dome-shaped muscle located between the chest cavity, which holds your heart and lungs, and the abdominal cavity, which holds your stomach and intestines. In normal breathing, the diaphragm contracts when you breathe in. This enlarges the chest cavity and creates a partial vacuum that draws air into the lungs. When the diaphragm relaxes, this vacuum vanishes and air flows out of the lung as the elastic fibers throughout the lungs contract.

The nose is a very effective air conditioner (see p. 40). Hairs at the opening of the nose (nostrils) trap large particles of dust. Mucus, a special fluid produced by glands in the nose, traps fine particles. Hair-like structures, called cilia, move the dirty mucus out of the nose. At the same time that air is being cleaned, it is also being warmed to a temperature of about 95° Fahrenheit. Air is also hu-

Oxygen Exchange in the Air Sacs

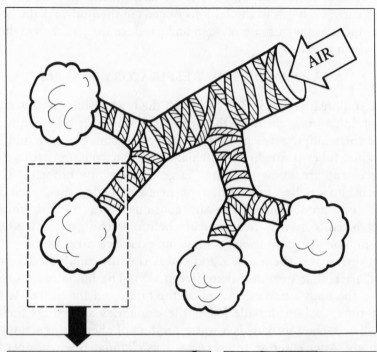

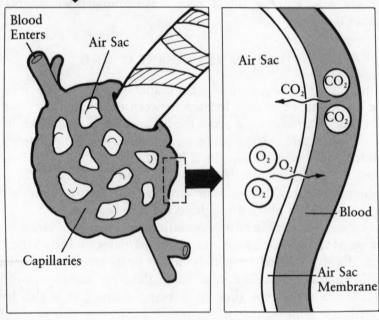

Main Breathing Muscle: Diaphragm

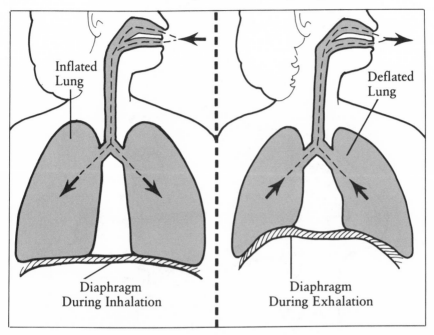

midified as it moves past the turbinates which protrude into the nasal cavity. By the time it reaches the trachea, inspired air has a humidity of about 97 percent.

The lining of the nasal cavity and of the lung's air passages is similar. The humidifying, warming, and cleaning process continues as air flows through the bronchi and bronchioles (see p. 41). Mucus-producing glands and goblet cells manufacture a thin film of sticky fluid which traps irritant particles. Tiny hairs (cilia) on the ends of the cells lining the bronchioles gently sweep the particle-laden mucus toward the pharynx. From there the material is either swallowed or coughed out.

What is Asthma?

Asthma is a chronic illness in which the bronchioles, or small windpipes, are "twitchy" or overreact compared to those of the aver-

Air Conditioner: Nasal Passage

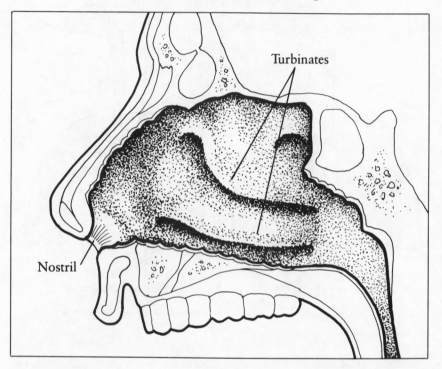

age person. The bronchioles become temporarily narrowed or blocked when they overreact in response to various triggers or stimuli. The tendency to overreact is often present from infancy. Parents with asthma may pass this tendency on to some of their children. Most children with asthma symptoms have a mild form of the disease and, if properly treated, find it more of a nuisance than a tragedy.

Asthma is known by many names including wheezy bronchitis, asthmatic bronchitis and bronchial asthma. It is often misdiagnosed as pneumonia. Doctors describe it as reversible obstructive airway disease (ROAD). This indicates that the narrowing of the bronchioles is temporary.

How do the bronchioles become narrowed or blocked? The bronchioles become blocked three different ways during an asthma attack. The muscles encircling a bronchiole tighten and thus narrow the air passage.

Fluid and cells enter the lining of the bronchioles. This causes the lining to swell and narrows the air passage still further. Mucous glands in the bronchiole secrete more mucus than usual. This mucus narrows the windpipe even more and can block the remaining opening in the bronchiole.

What is an asthma attack? An asthma attack is any episode or flare of asthma in which worsening of breathing interrupts ongoing activities or requires some intervention such as rest or medicine, be-

Air Cleaner: Cilia and Mucous Glands

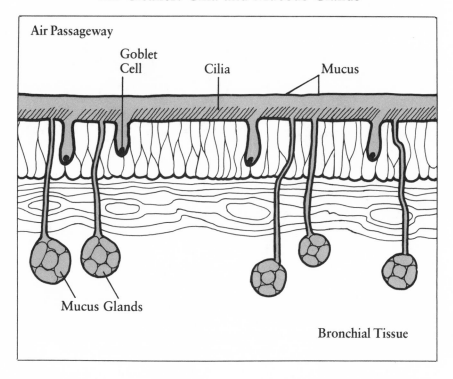

Air Passageway

Goblet Cell

Cilia

Mucus

Mucus Glands

Bronchial Tissue

fore one can resume normal and comfortable breathing. Such narrowing of the bronchioles can be set off by any number of triggers. The terms episode, flare, problem and attack are similar. I use the term attack infrequently since it implies a sudden, dramatic and unpredictable onset. An asthma episode usually develops slowly and gives plenty of warning to the knowledgeable parent.

What are some of the triggers of an asthma episode? In children, viral respiratory infections, such as colds and bronchitis, are the most common triggers of an asthma episode. Bacterial sinus infections may trigger a flare. Exercise, especially in cold air, often sets

Normal Bronchiole

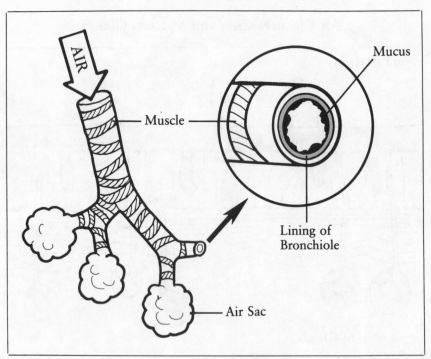

Exterior view shows muscle encircling bronchiole. Cross-section shows normal thickness of muscle, bronchiole lining and mucus.

off an episode of asthma. Irritants such as cigarette smoke, perfumes, dust and chemicals, also trigger asthma. Allergens, substances that are capable of producing allergic responses or symptoms, are significant triggers in five to ten percent of our patients. These include house dust, pollens, molds, animal dander and some foods. Emotional upsets indirectly trigger an episode when they lead to an outburst of yelling, crying, screaming or laughing. These activities themselves can provoke an attack.

Does every episode need treatment? In general, yes. The severity

Bronchiole During Flare

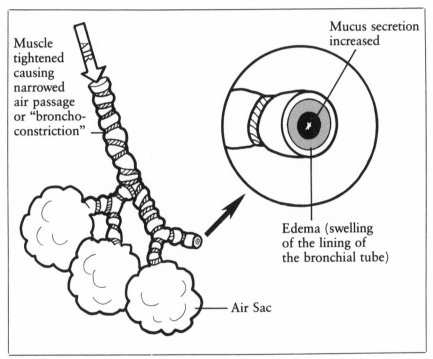

Exterior view shows narrowed bronchioles and over-inflated alveoli. Cross-section shows narrowed bronchiole almost blocked by swollen lining and increased mucus.

of a flare is not predictable at the outset. Medications are less effective as the episode gains momentum. Early treatment leads to the best result. Treatment should be based on your knowledge of your child's previous pattern and your assessment of the current episode.

Diagnosing and Naming Asthma

In most cases asthma can be suspected by a physician who pays close attention to the story of a child's symptoms. These often include coughing, wheezing, and previous bouts of bronchitis or pneumonia. When examination shows two of the four signs of asthma trouble—wheezing, the chest skin is sucked in, breathing out takes longer and the breathing rate is faster—the diagnosis of asthma is highly likely. The diagnosis becomes almost certain if these signs improve after the child inhales an adrenergic drug (see p. 73). A twenty percent increase in the peak flow rate (see p. 96) following the inhalation of an adrenergic drug can also confirm the diagnosis.

About 100,000 children in the United States are hospitalized each year with a diagnosis of acute bronchitis, an inflammation of the large airways, or bronchiolitis, an inflammation of the smaller airways. These diseases are caused by viruses. It is sometimes difficult for a physician to distinguish between these viral infections and asthma. Bronchitis caused by a virus may trigger an asthma episode. An asthma medication which dilates the bronchioles will improve the condition of a child with asthmatic bronchitis but will have little effect on a patient with acute bronchitis since this child's airways are not constricted. Thus a trial of asthma medicine may be a good way to clarify the diagnosis.

When an infant is ill and has rapid respirations his or her problem is often diagnosed as pneumonia. Frequently the correct diagnosis is asthma or bronchiolitis. Twenty-five years ago, it was thought that children younger than twelve months of age did not have enough muscle around their bronchioles to produce the narrowing which causes asthma symptoms. We now know that they do. However, some infants do not wheeze with an asthma episode. The only way to find out whether asthma treatment will help these young children is to try it. Even a three-month-old child with asthma will benefit from asthma medicine.

Some physicians recognize the symptoms of asthma and treat it with proper medications. However in order to spare the parents worry they don't use the word asthma. Instead, they describe the situation as a "wheezing problem." Of course, if you are not told your child has asthma you are being deprived of the opportunity to learn about it. You can't discuss the problem with friends whose children have asthma. You can't find a book in the library about "wheezing problems." If your doctor doesn't tell you your child has asthma, you will not be able to take care of the next asthma episode any better than the first.

The Four Signs of Asthma Trouble

LEARN THEM TO KEEP YOUR CHILD OUT OF THE EMERGENCY ROOM AND HOSPITAL

Asthma causes more hospital admissions and more emergency room visits than any other chronic illness of childhood. Most of these traumatic events can be avoided if you have the skill to accurately observe the four signs of asthma trouble: wheezing, the chest skin is sucked in, breathing out takes longer, and the breathing rate is faster. You must also have a written plan, worked out in advance with your doctor, that tells when to start or add medicine. The four signs can be monitored through the course of an asthma episode. If the medicine produces significant improvement, then you can relax. If not, it is time to add another medicine or see the doctor—according to your pre-set plan.

The four signs of asthma trouble

- Wheezing
- Chest skin is sucked in
- Breathing out takes longer
- Breathing is faster

Wheezing: This is the high-pitched, whistling sound that occurs when air flows through narrowed bronchioles. At the start of an attack the wheezing occurs only when the child is breathing out (expiration). In mild cases you can only hear wheezing with a stethoscope or with your ear against the chest. As the symptoms worsen the wheezing becomes louder and may also occur when the child breathes in. If many bronchioles become totally blocked, the decrease in airflow results in less wheezing. The absence of wheezing in a child with severe retractions and prolonged expiration is a sign of serious trouble. When this patient improves and the bronchioles start to open, wheezing will reappear.

Chest skin is sucked in (retractions): The soft tissues of the chest wall are sucked in when your child cannot draw air into the lungs fast enough. As the chest cavity expands, these tissues are sucked in by negative pressure. You will notice that the tissue between the ribs, above the breastbone and above the collarbone may be sucked in. Retractions may be an early sign of an asthma episode in an infant. This sign is much more obvious in slim children than in chubby children. Some slim children suck in their chest skin a little bit when they are breathing normally. Learn your child's usual breathing pattern so that you can detect a change.

Breathing out takes longer than breathing in (in-to-out ratio): Ordinarily a child takes at least as long to breathe in as to breathe out. During an asthma flare, the outflow of air is blocked more than the inflow and breathing out takes longer. In a mild episode, the change may not be noticeable. In a moderate flare, breathing out may take twice as long as breathing in. In a severe flare, breathing out may take more than twice as long as breathing in.

See if you can notice the "in-out" rhythm in your own breathing. Then try to observe it when your child is breathing normally. Since it is hard to judge by looking alone try breathing in and out with your child to get the feel of the breathing pattern. Do this a few times while your child is well so that you are prepared to notice a change during an asthma flare.

Breathing faster: Most children breathe faster than usual when they have an asthma episode. To count the breathing rate, either count for a full minute or count for half a minute and multiply by two. In young children it is often easier to see the belly move in and out

Sucking in the Chest Skin: Retractions

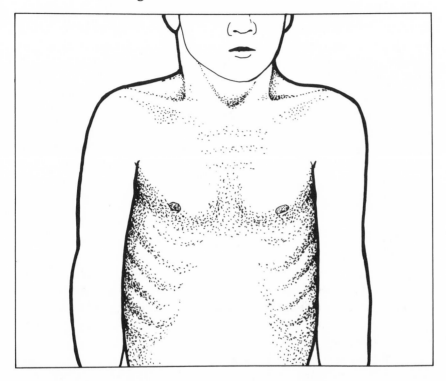

rather than to notice the chest move. Fast breathing is often the first sign of an asthma episode in an infant.

Normal breathing rates
per minute

Infants	25–60
1–4 yrs	20–30
5–14 yrs	15–25
14–18 yrs	11–23

A sleeping child usually breathes at a slower rate. If you know your child's usual rate you will be able to judge whether his breathing rate is becoming more normal with treatment. Occasionally an older child will have so much trouble breathing out that his breathing rate actually slows during a flare.

Any parent can learn the four signs of asthma trouble by watching the child during an asthma episode. With practice you will be able to notice whether each of the four trouble signs is improving or worsening as time passes. After a child has been treated in the office for a severe episode we ask the parents to record progress at home. If parents know how long it takes for each medication to work and how long the effect should last, they can decide whether progress is adequate or whether they should consult us for further advice.

Monitoring the Progress of an Asthma Episode

It is usually obvious when a child is having an asthma episode, but it is sometimes difficult to tell how serious a particular episode is. Older children will tell you how they feel and can compare it with previous occurrences. Younger children may just "not act themselves" and have trouble breathing.

When we evaluate a child who is having an asthma problem, we observe the four signs of asthma trouble as accurately as possible. These are described in the box below to help you grade the severity of each sign.

Mild asthma flares should almost always be treated, but many families can handle them at home alone or with telephone consultation. Persistence of even mild symptoms for several days should prompt a visit to the physician. Moderate flares should improve with usual treatments at home. You should have medications at home which will lead to significant improvement within two hours. If improvement does not occur you should consult your physician. Severe flares should be evaluated and treated in the doctor's office or emergency room.

Severity of the Four Trouble Signs

Severity	Wheezing	Sucking in chest skin	Breathing out longer	Breathing faster
Mild	barely noticeable	barely noticeable	out slightly longer	slight increase
Moderate	obvious throughout expiration	indentation obvious	out may be twice as long as in	up to 50% increase
Severe	inspiration and expiration	marked indentations	out more than twice as long	more than 50% above usual rate

Once you can judge the severity of a flare you can get phone advice from the physician on how to manage it. For example, when Ryan (see chapter one) had a problem late one night, his parents started treatment according to a pre-set plan. His dad called me at 9:00 A.M. to say that Ryan had improved. However he was still wheezing in and out, his breathing out was prolonged and he was breathing faster than usual. I advised him to come in for a treatment with a compressor-driven nebulizer in three hours if he did not improve significantly. At noon Mr. Parker called saying Ryan was wheezing less, his breathing in and out were equal and his respiratory rate had slowed down somewhat. He felt that Ryan was definitely better and continued to treat him at home.

Harriet Goodwin called one afternoon to say that Josh (see chapter one) had started a cold three days before, then developed a cough and had a slight expiratory wheeze. His in to out ratio was equal. He was taking full doses of theophylline and using a metaproterenol inhaler four times a day. She thought he should take a burst of prednisone and wanted to check with me before starting it. Based on her information I agreed that this was the next step.

Eighteen-month-old Dwayne came to the office one Saturday evening with his first episode of asthma. He was wheezing so loudly I could hear it across the room. His in-out ratio was equal, he had mild to moderate retractions, and he was breathing sixty times a minute. As I examined and treated him, I reviewed these findings with his parents. Fifteen minutes after I started treatment, the wheeze could only be heard with a stethoscope. His in-out ratio was unchanged, the retractions had lessened, and he was breathing forty times a minute. Since this flare was moderately severe I asked his parents whether they preferred to observe and treat Dwayne at home or to admit him to the hospital. They felt they could manage at home. When I called two hours later, his father reported a slight wheeze, no retractions, in-out ratio equal, and respirations at 48 per minute. He felt confident that Dwayne's condition was stable. I knew I could count on his father to monitor the situation until we met the next morning. He would call for help if Dwayne's symptoms worsened.

Keeping An Asthma Record

A daily record of symptoms, medications, and comments has helped me to improve the status of many children with asthma (see p. 68). On entering a new practice ten years ago, I found that almost all of my patients with asthma were having problems that could be avoided with aggressive treatment. Some coughed only at night, some wheezed with exercise, and others seemed to develop severe asthma flares without warning. Parents usually did not know which triggers provoked an asthma episode in their child. They did not understand the relationship between the dose of a drug and its effects, both good and bad. I spent the greater part of each office visit trying to determine the effects of various triggers and medications on the symptoms of the child with asthma. The parents' recollections were neither complete nor precise.

To improve recall, I devised a record for the parent or older child to keep on a daily basis. Now parents collect data in advance and we spend the office visit *analyzing* what happened rather than trying to remember the facts. I can usually make informed suggestions for adjusting medications based on the asthma record.

Wheezing, cough, interference with activities, and sleep are rated on a daily basis. Each dose of medicine is listed as is the peak flow rate. This record has enabled parents to:

- recall accurately the events since the last visit by providing a structured format
- communicate clearly and succinctly on the telephone
- learn when to start medication
- learn when to reduce medication
- compare the effects of various dosages and combinations of medications
- remember to give medication
- identify triggers which regularly provoke an episode
- reduce the length and thus the cost of a visit
- determine the pattern of their child's episodes
- become responsible for treatment
- record and analyze peak flow data

The parents are in charge of seeing that the child takes enough medication to be normally active without developing symptoms. Recording the day's symptoms and level of activity helps parents tune in to their child's condition.

Parents keep a daily record while they are learning about asthma. After they have a good understanding of what is going on with their child's asthma they keep the record only during times of difficulty.

A fourteen-year-old girl came to the office because of frequent cough that had continued for six days. She had no history of asthma. On exam she coughed every fifteen seconds and could not take a deep breath without coughing. The mean peak flow for children of her height was 480 liters per minute. Her best effort was 320. After three whiffs of metaproterenol, spaced two minutes apart, she felt better and her peak flow increased to 380, almost twenty percent.

I made a diagnosis of asthma and prescribed a double whiff of metaproterenol four times a day and 200 mg of theophylline every twelve hours. After three days she increased the theophylline to 300 mg every twelve hours. When I saw her a week later she coughed only once during a fifteen minute visit. She was cheerful, her lungs were clear as before and her peak flow was 460.

Her asthma record demonstrates:

- wakefulness due to theophylline on the first day of treatment

Asthma Record: teenager

Date	Wheeze	Cough	Activity	Night	Inhaled Adrenergic	Theophylline	Comments
11/3	0	2	3	3	✓✓ / ✓✓	200 / 200	Feel like drank coffee — Couldn't sleep.
11/4	0	1	3	2	✓✓ / ✓✓	200 / 200	Coughed more after 2 p.m.
11/5	0	1	3	1	✓✓ / ✓✓	200 / 200	felt pretty good — only slight cough.
11/6	0	1	1	0	✓✓ / ✓✓	300 / 300	worked outside — coughed more.
11/7	0	1	1	0	✓✓ / ✓✓	300 / 300	very tired afternoon.
11/8	0	1	1	0	✓✓ / ✓✓	300 / 300	felt good — a little trouble in gym
11/9	0	1	0	0	✓✓ / ✓✓	300 / 300	

- clear improvement after the dose of theophylline was increased on fourth day
- symptoms increase with exercise

Without a written record, it would have been impossible to remember the changes in cough, activity, and sleeping in this much detail. This teenager learned about her medication and her asthma by producing and analyzing her asthma record.

Mike, a six-year-old boy with a long history of asthma, came to the office because he had a cold for one week and a cough for several days. The exam showed some wheezing and a reduced peak flow rate. I prescribed long-acting theophylline every twelve hours, metaproterenol syrup every six hours and a metaproterenol inhaler. His mother phoned with a progress report three days later, stating that he had no wheeze or cough and that his activity and sleeping were

Asthma Record: six-year old

Date	Wheeze	Cough	Activity	Night	Inhaled Adrenergic	Theophylline	Metaproterenol
11/15	1	2	3	1	✓✓	✓✓	✓✓
11/16	0	1	1	0	0	✓✓	✓✓ ✓✓
11/17	0	0	0	0		✓✓	✓✓ ✓✓
11/18	0	0	0	0		✓✓	0
11/19	0	0	0	0		✓✓	

now normal. She had used the inhaler for only one day and discontinued metaproterenol by mouth after two days. We decided to give only one dose of theophylline the next day and then stop. Mike remained asymptomatic after medication was discontinued.

Early Clues

Once a parent knows how to evaluate an asthma flare, it is time to learn how to start treatment early. There are early clues that a problem is brewing. These will often be noticeable hours or even a day before the appearance of the obvious signs of wheezing, retraction, prolonged expiration, and increased breathing rate. Early clues are not always definite signs that an asthma episode is in the works, but they should make you think about the possibility. They can be grouped as changes in mood, changes in facial appearance, changes in breathing, verbal complaints and others.

Mood changes to watch for include anything that is different from the child's normal behavior. He or she may become aggressive or quiet; overactive, grouchy or tired; easily upset, nervous or sad; mopey or grumpy.

Facial appearance may change. The child's face may either be red or pale or look swollen. Dark circles under the eyes or increased perspiration are other clues.

Breathing changes include coughing, breathing through the mouth, or shortness of breath.

Verbal complaints may concern a tight chest, a hurting chest, a feeling that the child's chest is filling up, shortness of breath, fatigue, headache or a dry mouth. A child might say that his or her neck "feels funny" or maybe that he or she just doesn't feel well. Individual children may have some other complaint that can come to be seen as a forewarning of an asthma flare.

Other clues are yawning or an itchy chin or neck. Some young children stroke their necks in response to this itchy feeling. You may notice that some other mannerism, not mentioned here, may foretell an asthma episode in your child.

It takes a while to tune in to these changes. Each child has his or her own set of early clues that you will learn to recognize as time goes on. This is particularly important if your child is under four years of age and too young to use a peak flow meter.

Triggers

The most common triggers (substances or events) which provoke asthma episodes are exercise, viral respiratory infections, irritants, cold air, allergens and mechanical events, such as coughing, yelling or laughing. Emotional events can be indirect triggers of asthma (see p. 62).

Overreactivity (hyperreactivity or sensitivity) of the airways varies greatly from person to person. Some children develop symptoms of asthma only after contact with a specific trigger. A very reactive child may have an asthma episode with each of the triggers mentioned above. The episode may be worsened by the presence of several triggers at the same time. Some children have an asthma episode only when several triggers occur simultaneously, such as exercise or exposure to smoke during a viral respiratory infection.

Individuals Vary in Their Reaction to each Trigger

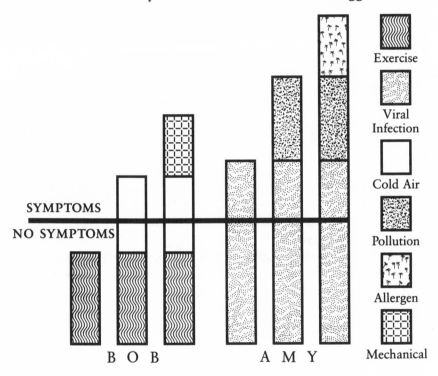

Bob has mildly reactive airways. Exercise alone will not trigger an attack, but exercise in cold air will. Laughing will worsen his symptoms. Amy is very sensitive to a number of triggers and gets an attack with a viral infection or exposure to a pollutant or to a cat. Triggers have an additive effect. Amy will have a worse asthma flare if she is exposed to several triggers at the same time.

Viral Infections

Viral respiratory infections are the most common trigger of asthma flares in young children. In this situation, the virus invades some part of the respiratory system. This can be the nose, the throat, the sinuses, any part of the airway (trachea, bronchi, bronchioles) as well as the lung tissue itself.

Viruses cause the air passages to narrow and to increase their reactivity in several different ways. They cause certain cells in the airway to release chemical mediators (histamine, leukotrienes and others). These mediators produce swelling (inflammation) of the lining of the bronchioles and thus narrow the air passages. These chemicals also cause an increase in mucus secretion. The mucus blocks the flow of air through the bronchioles. A viral infection may also reduce the number and sensitivity of special areas in the airways (beta-agonist receptor sites) that control bronchodilation.

You can reduce your child's exposure to viruses, but it is a major undertaking. We do not recommend that a child be kept at home to prevent exposure to viruses. However, it would make sense to keep the child who gets severe asthma episodes away from playmates who are sick with a viral respiratory infection. We also recommend influenza vaccine as a preventive measure for all children who take asthma medicine daily and also for those children who have severe asthma episodes, even if they only occur two or three times a year.

Antibiotic medicines such as penicillin, amoxicillin and erythromycin cannot kill viruses. Therefore, these medications are of no help in the treatment of asthma episodes triggered by a virus infection.

Exercise

Exercise is the most common trigger of asthma. Eighty percent of people with asthma get some degree of chest tightness, cough, or wheeze when they exercise. These symptoms usually mean that their asthma is inadequately controlled.

Asthma should not limit the activity of any child who is receiving proper treatment. The toddler should be able to run around outside.

The gradeschooler can participate fully in all gym class and recess activities. High school students can pick any sport they want. Obviously, if a child is in the the middle of an asthma episode, his or her ability to exercise will be limited. Ordinarily the student will be back to normal activity within a week.

Often a child with asthma triggered by exercise will restrict physical activity almost automatically. One father was totally unaware that his son limited his activity. He was surprised to hear his son tell me that he plays goalie in soccer because he gets a tight chest or starts wheezing after a few minutes in a more active position. Limitation is all right if it is necessary. However, in almost every instance, children with asthma can exercise without discomfort if a proper treatment plan is followed.

Our patients compete in hockey, soccer, cross-country running, basketball, and tennis at a varsity level. Three of eight players on the first-place basketball team in a league in Amherst, Massachusetts, have asthma. Several years ago, a mother caught me between periods at a game. She wanted me to know that since her son started using an adrenergic drug by inhaler before games he could play a full game. The year before he had had to quit at half-time.

Because we believe that the child with well-controlled asthma can participate in every sport, we do not steer our patients to swimming. We want them to play the sport they enjoy the most and are good at. After all, Bill Koch, who won an Olympic silver medal in cross country skiing, has asthma. He used adequate medication to protect against the dual triggers of exercise and cold air.

Swimming is the competitive sport which doctors recommend most frequently to children with asthma. Because it requires exertion of short duration that takes place at the proper temperature and humidity, it rarely triggers an asthma episode. Baseball, football, and gymnastics also do not require a high level of sustained exertion. Still, we say let the child, not the doctor, pick the sport. No sport will cause symptoms if the athlete and the physician have worked out a good treatment plan.

Some researchers now believe that exercise triggers asthma by lowering the temperature of the bronchioles as air is exchanged rapidly. Hyperventilation without exercise can also cause asthma symptoms.

Exercise-induced asthma is a term applied to asthma in which symptoms only occur *after at least five minutes of sustained exercise.* Symptoms of exercise-induced asthma usually disappear within two hours if lung function was normal before the exercise. Therefore, treatment is much briefer than for an episode of asthma provoked by a viral respiratory infection.

To prevent exercise-induced asthma:

• Warm the air by breathing through the nose (a natural air conditioner and warmer). One can create a reservoir of warm air by wearing a painter's or surgeon's mask covered by a scarf when out in cold weather.

• Use an adrenergic drug or cromolyn by inhaler fifteen minutes before exercise. Fast-release theophylline taken an hour before exercise may also protect against a flare.

Remember, asthma symptoms that come on after less than five minutes of exercise are a sign that a child's asthma is inadequately treated.

Environment

Environmental factors frequently trigger asthma episodes. However, most parents do not have to tear their house apart in order to provide a healthy living situation for their child with asthma. The vigor of environmental controls should match the severity of the asthma problem. If your child has mild asthma, you should prohibit smoking in the house. If your child's asthma is well controlled, no further changes are necessary. If not, consider taking additional steps to minimize environmental triggers.

Some common *irritants* are cigarette smoke, dust, deodorants, perfume, paint, and overhumidified air. They affect everyone's ability to breathe, but children with asthma often have a more severe reaction to them. Fumes from car exhausts and smoke from factory chimneys or burning leaves can also trigger a flare.

If you *smoke a cigarette,* a cigar or a pipe in the house, do not think for a moment that you are not hurting your child. Children with asthma wheeze longer and more often if someone smokes in the house—anywhere in the house. We have never told a parent to quit smoking. We only ask that they not smoke in the house or in any enclosed space, such as the car, if their child has asthma.

House dust can be both an irritant and an allergen. Invisible particles of house dust come from the disintegration of rugs, mattresses, stuffed toys, the skin of pets and the bodies and feces of house mites and cockroaches. They float in the air and fall all around. If your child has chronic asthma (takes medication daily) or seems to have difficulty breathing on exposure to dust, you should make some effort to decrease the dust in the environment.

Since your child spends more time in the bedroom than any other room, your effort should be concentrated there.

To Reduce Bedroom Dust

1. Keep books, toys, knick-knacks and other dust-collecting objects to a minimum.
2. Vacuum carpets weekly and shampoo them occasionally.
3. Wipe woodwork, closets and drawers daily with a damp rag.
4. Launder curtains frequently. Avoid heavy curtains.
5. Store only this season's clothes in the closet. Keep door closed.
6. Seal hot-air vents in homes with tape or cover them with five or six layers of cheesecloth.
7. Replace or clean furnace filters each month during the winter.
8. Encase mattress and box spring in a mite-proof, airtight cover.
9. Consider carpet and curtain removal, air filtration, and cleaning of heating ducts if patient's condition does not improve with these simple measures.

Adapted from "Allergic and Irritant Triggers of Asthma" by Mark Holbreich in *Manual of Clinical Problems in Asthma, Allergy and Related Disorders.* Don A. Bukstein, M.D. and Robert C. Strunk, M.D., eds. Little, Brown and Company, 1984. Used with permission.

Any odor or fume may cause symptoms. Your child should stay away from hair sprays, perfumes, paints, and scented soaps if they have caused any breathing difficulty in the past. Sometimes cooking odors and smoke cause an asthma episode. A vent in the kitchen would reduce this possibility.

Room air should be a comfortable *temperature*. Cold air may trigger an asthma episode. Hot air dries the mucus produced in the windpipes and interferes with normal cleansing of the airway.

The ideal *humidity* is between 25 and 40 percent. This allows enough moisture for the cilia to perform their cleaning activities. Air with a higher moisture content may act as an irritant and may also promote the growth of molds and mites. A humidification system can be built into your forced air heating system. A free standing ultrasonic humidifier will maintain humidity at the desired level. To control the moisture level most effectively use a device that has a humidistat.

If your home is heated by a forced air system, you can replace the standard filters in the system with an electrostatic air precipitator, which acts as an *air cleaner*. Central electrostatic air precipitators are available from airconditioning distributers or heating contractors at about $600. Various free-standing filtering systems are available for use in houses heated by electricity or hot water. One of the most effective systems is the high-energy particulate air (HEPA) filter. A HEPA room unit costs about $300–500; free-standing electrostatic air precipitators are less expensive. Either can be purchased from stores that sell respiratory therapy equipment.

Wood stoves create a special problem for children with asthma because of the smoke they draw into the house. As hot air, filled with smoke, rises up the chimney, cold air is drawn from the rest of the house into the stove. This air is replaced by outside air containing the smoke that has just left the chimney. Thus, even a tight wood stove draws sooty air into the home. To solve this problem, your stove should burn hot to ensure a more complete burning and less smoke. Attach a catalytic converter to cut smoke and pollution further.

Allergy and Allergy Shots

■

EMLEN JONES, M.D.

Allergy is an acquired hypersensitivity to a foreign substance (allergen). Symptoms are caused by an antibody reaction which takes place in the body on exposure to the allergen. Frequently, this reaction can be confirmed by a positive skin test to the offending substance. Important common allergens include pollens from trees, grasses or weeds, animal danders, dusts and molds.

Asthma is not an allergy. However, allergy does play a significant role in five to ten percent of children with asthma. Children whose asthma episodes are consistently related to exposure to a specific substance (for example, dogs, grasses, hay or dust) are likely to have an allergic trigger. The same is true for children who have hay fever or eczema or develop asthma symptoms at the same time each spring or summer.

Why should we find out if an allergy provokes some of the child's asthma symptoms? Mainly, to advise the child to avoid the allergen if he or she can. The same philosophy applies to any other trigger of asthma. Also, some children and adolescents may benefit from allergy shots (immunotherapy). Several studies have confirmed the benefit of allergy shots in appropriately selected patients with asthma.

Which children should be investigated for the presence of allergy? We would suggest testing any child who requires asthma medication daily for three or more months of the year, even in the absence of an allergic history. This testing may identify specific allergic triggers which could be avoided.

Testing should also be done on any child who has intermittent asthma and, in addition, a history that suggests either a reaction to specific allergens, or allergic symptoms such as hay fever or eczema, or a strong family history of allergies.

How is allergy investigated? A detailed history which includes family and environmental details is taken. This is followed by a careful physical exam to look for any signs of allergy. Laboratory studies usually include a blood count and measurement of IgE, an antibody associated with allergy. Various other tests are done in specific circumstances. Finally, skin tests are performed. Small amounts of suspected allergens are either pricked, scratched on, or injected into the skin and the local reaction is observed.

Not long ago allergy shots were overused in the treatment of asthma. The advent of more effective drug treatment has limited their use. We recommend allergy shots (immunotherapy), for children who show significant asthma symptoms to allergens that cannot be avoided. Approximately twelve of our 400 patients with asthma take allergy shots. If allergy shots are started, they should be continued for a minimum of two years before deciding whether or not they are helpful. Shots are not given for an allergen which can be avoided, for example, a pet. The shots do not replace standard treatments for asthma but are given in addition to them.

Emotions

Asthma is caused by a complex set of physiological reactions which are not yet completely understood. We can say for sure, however, that asthma is not due to a defective mother-child relationship or to any other psychological problem as has been suggested in the past. What role, then, do the emotions play in asthma?

Though emotional factors do not cause asthma they can affect the person with asthma in several ways:

The expression of emotions by laughing, crying or yelling can stimulate the vagus nerve. This may cause the muscles around the bronchioles to tighten and may trigger wheezing, especially in a child with pre-existing unstable airways. Consider this scenario—a ten-year-old boy gets into an argument with his mother about doing the dishes. She scolds him and he runs out of the house yelling at her. A few minutes later he is wheezing. Did the emotions cause this asthma episode? Indirectly they did, since an emotional event generated two triggers: mechanical (yelling) and exercise (running). If this same boy were acting in a play and had to yell and run, he would start to wheeze even though no emotions were involved.

Anxiety during a flare may produce hyperventilation—excessive rate and depth of breathing—which can worsen the attack.

Anxiety can cause one person with asthma to assign greater importance to a symptom than would another.

Patients with chronic asthma sometimes become angry and frustrated and rebel against taking their medications, thus worsening their situation.

Some children find that they get special attention when they have an asthma episode. If the benefits outweigh the unpleasantness of an episode, these children may consciously or unconsciously change the way they breathe. Only two of our four hundred patients with asthma seem to have consciously or unconsciously decided that the attention is worth the discomfort.

The ability to relax may shorten an episode.

What is the effect of asthma on the child's emotions? If a child's asthma is well controlled, as it should be for ninety-nine percent of children, asthma should play little or no role in his or her psychic functioning. Children with asthma have as many different personality types as children without asthma.

We find that children who develop asthma while they are patients in our pediatric practice have little difficulty adjusting to it. Since we rarely give epinephrine shots, children and parents do not delay treatment for fear of them. Parents learn how to treat asthma early and aggressively at home. The treatment is painless, and the surroundings are pleasant. Some of our patients require daily treatment with three or four medicines, yet they lead active lives and play competitive sports.

If asthma is not well-controlled, the effects on a child's psyche may be serious indeed. Most hospital emergency rooms are not geared to the care of children. It may take weeks to recover psychologically from a single emergency room visit (see the "Thanksgiving Disaster," p. 185). A hospital stay may have worse effects, though not necessarily so. We expect a parent to stay with the child under ten years of age twenty-four hours a day if his or her other responsibilities allow.

Some children enter our practice after having been subjected to years of poorly-controlled asthma, punctuated by hospital admissions and numerous trips to the emergency room. Often they and their parents appear as dependent, helpless individuals who are terrified of or resigned to the next asthma episode. They have little or no understanding of asthma as a process or what they can and should do about it. Over a period of several years of education and support, most of these children and their parents learn how to manage their asthma episodes and in the process become more confident, outgoing individuals.

Other Triggers

Cold air: It causes the bronchioles to become more reactive. The exact cause for this is unknown. In order to warm the winter air, one can construct a face mask for a snow suit. One mother sewed a piece of flannel to one side of the snow suit hood and made a velcro fastener for the other side. This mask creates a reservoir of warm air which can be rebreathed.

The Air Warmer

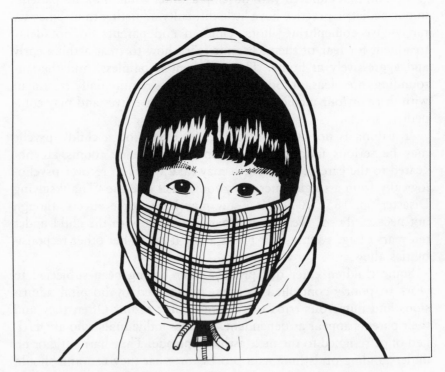

Mechanical triggers: Certain activities such as laughing, crying, yelling, and coughing stimulate the vagus nerve which leads to the lungs. When stimulated this nerve may cause bronchoconstriction that varies with the degree of instability of the child's bronchioles.

Weather: When the weather changes, asthma often flares. This is usually due to an indirect effect rather than a change in barometric pressure. A weather change may bring cold air or the wind may blow in irritants or pollens from a distant source. A thermal inversion may cause increased air pollution. Each of these is a trigger in its own right.

Coughing

Children who cough at night, cough with exercise, cough in polluted areas and have other symptoms of asthma such as wheezing or a tight chest with exercise are easy to diagnose. Coughing at night or with exercise usually indicates that a child's asthma is inadequately treated. In many children a cough is often the first sign of an asthma episode. The typical asthma cough is usually short, high pitched, and non-productive. It may occur steadily several times per minute.

A child who has had a cough for more than two weeks may have asthma even though no wheezing is present. We measure the child's ability to breathe out quickly (the peak expiratory flow rate) to check for this possibility. If the peak flow increases twenty percent after an inhaled bronchodilator is given, we diagnose the child as having asthma and start treatment.

In a mild variant form, asthma produces a cough, but no shortness of breath or wheezing. Physicians who study asthma have found that some children who have a cough for many weeks have entirely normal physical examinations and normal lung function tests. Many of these children may completely lose their coughs when they take standard asthma medication, but begin to cough again after medication is stopped. They are diagnosed as having "cough variant asthma."

Factors which make this diagnosis more likely are a history of allergic respiratory conditions in the family, bronchiolitis (inflammation of the small bronchioles) in infancy, previous episodes of bronchitis, or pneumonia, or a tendency to prolonged chest colds.

We often recommend that a child who has a cough of long duration that interferes with sleep or activity be given a trial of treatment with theophylline. We do this even if the child shows no significant increase in peak flow after inhaling a bronchodilator. If he or she improves with treatment the diagnosis of cough variant asthma is confirmed. Many of these children develop additional symptoms of asthma over time. In that case the "cough variant" name no longer applies since it refers only to children who have coughing as their only asthma symptom.

Natural Course of Asthma in Children
■

EMLEN H. JONES, M.D.

Each person has his or her own pattern of asthma both for individual episodes and over a span of years. The tendency to have overreactive airways lasts a lifetime. However, most people do not exhibit symptoms after the teen years. An individual may have an episode after years of being symptom-free if he is subjected to an unusually potent trigger or set of triggers.

The severity of episodes or presence of symptoms often decreases with age for several reasons. The diameter of the bronchioles increases dramatically from young infancy to early childhood. As a result, the reaction to an asthma trigger may no longer block air flow significantly. Respiratory infections are not as frequent in older children as they are in preschoolers. Finally, certain viruses which trigger asthma damage the bronchial tree at a site which is more vulnerable in infants and younger children than in older children or adults.

It is impossible to predict with accuracy the long-term course of asthma symptoms in an individual. Some general statements can be made based on research here and abroad. However, these studies vary greatly in their definition of asthma and its severity in their subjects. Several large studies in Great Britain give us the following information. Most asthma starts in childhood. At least three percent and maybe as many as eleven percent of children have asthma symptoms at some time. Most of these children (eighty-five percent) have mild asthma which can be easily controlled. Fifty percent of children stop wheezing completely by adulthood. However, symptoms can recur at any time of life. Most who are still wheezing as adults have milder symptoms.

The conclusions of research studies are varied and sometimes contradictory. Some researchers have found that children who develop asthma after six months of age and who do not have significant allergies are very likely to outgrow their asthma symptoms. In another study sixty percent of the children who developed asthma before age sixteen were symptom-free eleven years later compared to thirty percent of those who developed it after age sixteen.

Other studies have demonstrated that children whose asthma is triggered primarily by upper respiratory infections and who improve between four and six years of age are less likely to have asthma symptoms in the future than children who have continuous asthma symptoms or significant allergies. The participants in most of these studies did not have the benefit of present-day treatment. Whether such therapy affects long-term outcome is unknown.

What about severe problems? Death from an acute attack is extremely rare. Only one out of every 25,000 children with asthma will die of it this year. Improved medications and techniques for home management should make hospitalization unusual. However, a child with severe asthma may be hospitalized several times. Though severe asthma does not usually cause chronic lung disease, lung damage can occur with cigarette smoking or in high air pollution areas.

Asthma Record—Please bring at each visit

Many things can *trigger* an asthma flare including colds or infections, exercise, irritants, allergens, and cold air. *Note any trigger which seems to affect your child the day it occurs. Can you detect any early warning signs before* wheezing occurs? Most common are: cough, sneezing, scratchy throat, itchy neck, grumpiness.

Date	Wheeze	Cough	Activity	Night	Inhaled Adrenergic	Theophylline	Prednisone	Cromolyn	Peak Flow			Comments

	0		1		2		3
Wheeze	None		Some		Medium		Severe
Cough	None		Occasional		Frequent		Continuous
Activity	Normal		Can run short distance		Can walk only		Missed school or stayed indoors
Night	Fine		Slept well slightly wheezy		Awake 2–3 times with wheeze		Bad night, awake most of the time

3
Medication

The indications and dosages of all the drugs in this book have been recommended in the medical literature and conform to the practice of asthma experts throughout the country. However, the information provided here is general and may not apply to your child's specific situation. DO NOT CHANGE YOUR CHILD'S MEDICATION ROUTINE WITHOUT YOUR DOCTOR'S APPROVAL.

It's easy to treat some problems. For a strep throat you just take penicillin three times a day for ten days. No decisions about what dose, how long or whether to use other drugs. And side effects from penicillin are not common.

Asthma treatment is different. The treatment routine should be tailored to the individual child and family. Your physician has four different medication groups to choose from:

Adrenergic drugs also known as beta-adrenergic, beta agonist, or adrenalin-type drugs are used to treat occasional asthma episodes.

Theophylline is used to treat occasional asthma episodes and as a long-term preventative medication.

Cromolyn, also known as cromolyn sodium, prevents asthma episodes—both as a long-term preventative treatment and as a short-term preventative measure before exercise or exposure to allergens.

Steroids, also known as cortico-steroids, have several uses. Oral preparations are commonly given in a short burst to treat a severe episode. Inhaled steroids are used daily to prevent episodes.

It often takes time to work out which medicines should be used for a particular child. The proper dose of medicine is usually determined after a period of trial and error. Your child's treatment must be adjusted, taking both symptoms and adverse effects into account.

This chapter outlines when medications should be used, how they affect the bronchioles, what trouble they can cause and the time factors that apply to each drug. There is guidance on when to start and when to stop treatment (see Home Treatment, chapter four, for further details). You will also find detailed instructions for using a metered dose inhaler since the instructions in the package insert are not adequate to provide optimal benefits to many users.

As a parent, you have the right and the responsibility to know what medicines are being prescribed for your child. In order to give medicine properly to your child, you need clear written instructions for each medication (see Medication Instructions, p. 123). You should be able to answer all of the following questions (adapted from Creer, 1986; see Resource List) before you leave the doctor's office:

- What is the name of this drug, and what is it supposed to do?
- Exactly when, and for how long, should my child take it?
- How long does it take for the medicine to start to work?
- What are the possible adverse effects?
- What should you do if it doesn't seem to be working?
- What should you do if you miss a dose by mistake?
- What should you do if you give an extra dose by mistake?
- Are there any medicines or foods that your child should not use while taking this drug?
- Is there an equally effective, but less expensive, form of this drug available?

It is important to take asthma medicine exactly as it is prescribed if it is to work correctly. If a medicine is prescribed for every six hours, that means every six hours, even if that dose falls in the middle of the night. If this routine is not convenient, be sure to let your physician know. He or she may be able to prescribe a long-acting form of the drug.

If you don't understand your doctor's directions, either you don't know enough about asthma and the medications used to treat it, or your physician is not giving you a logical explanation. Either situation is unsatisfactory. There is no room for guesswork or miscommunication in asthma. Never let the fear of asking a "stupid question" prevent you from clarifying an important point. There are no stupid questions when you are concerned about the medicine your child is taking. After you have read *Children With Asthma* several times, you should be able to understand any coherent explanation by a physician.

Adrenergic Drugs

Many physicians use an adrenergic drug as their first choice in the treatment of an asthma episode. These drugs dilate the bronchioles, making the air passages wider. They can be given by injection, taken by mouth or inhaled directly into the air passages.

Almost everyone who received emergency treatment for an asthma attack ten years ago remembers the epinephrine (adrenalin) shot. This shot causes bronchodilation and improves breathing within minutes. The effect lasts from two to ten hours depending on the preparation used. Side effects are pain on injection, anxiety, restlessness, shakiness, headache, and rapid, pounding, or irregular heart beat. In the past some children have been so afraid of getting an injection of epinephrine that they have not told their parents they were having an asthma problem. This led to a delay in treatment and a situation that was much more difficult to treat.

Now many physicians and emergency rooms give adrenergic drugs by compressor-driven nebulizer instead of using injections. This inhalation treatment is not painful. Also, because the drug goes directly to the bronchioles, a much smaller dose of medication is effective. Since the dose is small, adverse effects are less common and less severe than when the same drugs are given by injection or by mouth. The major disadvantage of this inhalation treatment is that it takes longer to administer and is thus more costly in terms of staff salaries. However, most parents can learn to use a compressor-driven nebulizer at home.

Adrenergic drugs can also be administered by a metered-dose inhaler (MDI) directly or through a holding chamber. Administration of adrenergic drugs by mouth is a simple and effective form of treatment for some children with mild asthma.

ADRENERGIC DRUGS BY INHALER

Adrenergic drugs taken by the inhaled route work more quickly and cause fewer side effects than any other medication used to treat an asthma episode. Many asthma specialists now use these drugs as their first-line treatment.

Metered dose inhalers (MDIs) are extremely useful but they have drawbacks. It is hard to learn the proper technique for using an inhaler. Once learned, this skill usually deteriorates if not monitored closely. Holding chambers can remedy this problem (see page 112). Finally, inhalers do not work well if they are dirty or if they are empty.

Selected Adrenergic Drugs for Inhalation

Generic names	Brand names
albuterol	Proventil, Ventolin
metaproterenol	Alupent, Metaprel
terbutaline	Brethaire

Indications:

- to treat mild, moderate and severe asthma flares
- to prevent bronchoconstriction due to exercise, cold and other triggers
- to relieve symptoms which come on suddenly
- to provide relief while the theophylline level is building up at the beginning of an episode

- to eliminate symptoms which are not controlled by a standard dose of theophylline, or when theophylline causes unacceptable side effects
- to open airways prior to using cromolyn if peak flow is not in green zone (see chapter four)

Desired effect: Relax smooth muscle around the bronchioles and allow them to open more completely.

Adverse effects: Throat discomfort, shakiness, rapid or pounding heartbeat, and nausea are common side effects which are not dangerous. An irregular heartbeat, chest pain, or any other symptom which concerns you or your child should be discussed with your doctor. Throat discomfort may be minimized by drinking water before inhaler use or by using a holding chamber (see p. 112).

Time factors: Begins to work within one to fifteen minutes. Effect should last about four to six hours. If it doesn't, your child's inhaler is dirty, empty, the technique is faulty, or the asthma is out of control and you should consult your physician.

Dosage: Two whiffs given at least two minutes apart every four to six hours while awake, as needed, up to four times a day. Waiting up to twenty minutes between whiffs may increase the effect. Some children get full relief with one whiff.

Comments: Since inhaled adrenergic medicines reach their peak effect in about sixty minutes, it is best to use the inhaler at least fifteen minutes before exercise.

The inhaler must be used correctly or it will provide little benefit. Technique should be reviewed at every visit to the doctor until it is perfect. After that, review technique every six to twelve months. Always bring your child's inhaler when you visit the doctor.

Instructions for Use of a Metered-Dose Inhaler

To use a metered-dose inhaler, your child should:

1. Put mouthpiece on the canister which contains the medicine.
2. Stand up.
3. Shake inhaler for two seconds.

Proper Inhaler Position

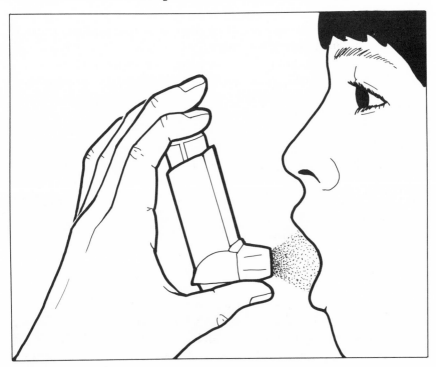

4. Position inhaler with canister (upside down) above mouthpiece.
5. Hold mouthpiece one to two inches from the lips and *open your mouth wide*. This position leads to more effective treatment because:
   - the parent can see the medication flowing into the mouth, indicating that timing and position are right.
   - it reduces the amount of medicine hitting the cheeks and palate because of turbulence on release.
6. Breathe out naturally, then
7. Open mouth wide and begin to inhale.
8. Squeeze canister down on mouthpiece and take about two to five seconds to inhale deeply.
9. Hold breath for as long as you can up to ten seconds.

10. Keep mouth open. If medicine floats out of your mouth, it didn't go deep enough. It is safe to repeat the dose without counting this one.

11. Wait at least two minutes. A twenty-minute wait may give better results but is often inconvenient.

12. Repeat steps 2 through 9. Most people benefit from this second inhalation. It delivers medicine into the bronchioles that have been opened by the first whiff.

Much of this information comes from Harper, 1981 (see p. 251).

Your child should feel better five minutes after using the inhaler and the effect should last for four to six hours. Do not use more than four double whiffs a day unless you check with your doctor. A child who needs to use the inhaler more often has an asthma problem which is deteriorating. Check with your doctor to see what additional treatment is needed.

CHECKLIST FOR MONITORING INHALER USE

We give our patients written and verbal instructions as well as a demonstration before they use the inhaler the first time. We observe the patient's technique and correct defects before he or she leaves the office. At the beginning of the next visit the child is asked to demonstrate its use. When we reviewed technique at a follow-up visit for twenty consecutive patients, we found that hardly anyone used the inhaler properly. So we designed a checklist for home use. We now try to review inhaler use each time the patient visits the office for any reason. Technique has improved and patients note that the effect of the inhaler lasts longer.

Check each line while observing inhaler technique. List can be used for several trials.

———————————Stand up

———————————Shake inhaler for two seconds

———————————Mouthpiece one to two inches from mouth

———————————Breathe out naturally

———————————Open mouth wide and inhale slowly for two to five seconds

—————————Keep mouth open
—————————Hold breath as long as you can up to ten seconds

Common errors are:

Inhalation is too fast: This leads to deposition of medicine on the throat, tongue, and palate instead of in the bronchioles.

Holds breath less than ten seconds: Medication leaves the bronchioles before it can settle to where it is needed.

No second inhalation: Not enough medication is delivered to the newly-expanded bronchioles.

Interval between whiffs is less than two minutes: Constricted windpipes block the passage of medication.

Is Your Inhaler Empty?

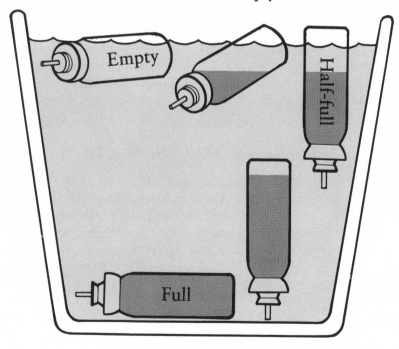

Your doctor can supply you with a practice inhaler. Since it contains propellant but no medicine, your child can practice several times without getting shaky. Timing is the biggest problem. Many people find it hard to pull air in at the exact time they release the medicine. Starting to breathe in slowly just before squeezing the canister may help your child draw the medicine in at the right time.

A mother told me she was concerned about her eleven-year-old, hockey-playing son. He had had to come off the ice three times in three weeks because of wheezing. This had not happened before. He ordinarily used an inhaler before practice and games. She did not think he was getting any benefit from his inhaler these days. I asked when he had cleaned it last. She said she thought it was last week but didn't know since that was his responsibility. Well, all it took was a little soap and water and he was back to his usual game.

A ten-year-old boy with mild asthma uses an inhaler as his sole medication to control wheezing. He mentioned that he was using it at bedtime but awakened with wheezing in the middle of the night and had to use it again. His asthma wasn't bad enough to cause that much trouble. On reviewing his inhaler technique, I found that he only used a single whiff. When he changed to a double whiff, he was able to sleep through the night.

A father with asthma thanked me for teaching him how to use the inhaler. Since he switched from the technique on the package insert to our instructions he gets more complete and sustained relief.

ADRENERGIC DRUGS BY MOUTH

We have found oral adrenergic drugs helpful in treating some children under three years of age. These children are too young to use a metered-dose inhaler. Older children can usually achieve the same benefit at a fraction of the dose by using the inhaled form of the drug. However, some children have no noticeable adverse effects from an oral preparation and find it more convenient to take than inhaled medication or theophylline.

Selected Adrenergic Drugs for Oral Use

Generic Names	Brand Names
albuterol	Proventil, Ventolin
metaproterenol	Alupent, Metaprel
terbutaline	Bricanyl, Brethine

Indications:

- a young child who has unacceptable side effects from theophylline and does not have a compressor-driven nebulizer at home
- a child who has fewer side effects from an adrenergic drug than theophylline and prefers the oral to the inhaled route of administration

Desired Effect: To relax smooth muscle around the bronchial tubes and allow them to open more completely.

Adverse Effects: Usually mild; shakiness, fast or pounding heartbeat, nausea.

Form:

- Liquid (albuterol 2 mg/5cc, metaproterenol 10 mg/5cc)
- Tablet (albuterol 2 and 4 mg, metaproterenol 10 and 20 mg, terbutaline 2.5 and 5 mg)

Time factors: The liquid or tablet takes thirty minutes to work and effect lasts about eight hours for albuterol and terbutaline and six hours for metaproterenol.

How to give: Usually given every six to eight hours around the clock.

Dosage: Initially we give albuterol liquid or tablet in a dose of 0.1 mg per kilogram every eight hours. We adjust the dose depending on the child's progress and the medication's side effects. The equivalent metaproterenol dose is 0.5 mg per kilogram every six hours. The *volume* of a starting dose for both medications is 2.5 cc for a twenty-two-pound child and 5.0 cc for a forty-four-pound child. The oral dose for each of these medications is several times as great as an equally effective inhaled dose.

Theophylline

Theophylline is a very useful drug for the treatment of mild and moderate asthma flares as well as a daily preventative medication. Many families find it convenient since the slow-release preparation often only needs to be given every twelve hours. A substantial number of children, however, have mild to moderate side effects of over-activity, upset stomach and headache. The dose must be carefully adjusted to minimize these effects. Often the combination of a low dose of theophylline and an inhaled adrenergic drug works better than either one alone.

Brand names: More than fifty, including Slo-bid, Theo-Dur, Quibron T/SR, Accubron, Constant-T, Elixophyllin, Slo-Phyllin, Somophyllin, and Theolair-SR

Indications:

• to treat mild or moderate asthma flare
• to prevent asthma symptoms

Desired Effect: To relax smooth muscle around the bronchial tubes and allow them to open more completely.

Adverse Effects: Most common are overactivity, nervousness, upset stomach, nausea, vomiting, loss of appetite, and headache. These effects are most prominent during the first few days. They may be avoided if treatment is started with a low dose and is increased gradually. Some slow-release preparations release theophylline more evenly and thus produce fewer adverse effects than fast-release forms.

There are many preparations of this drug. Some commonly used ones are listed in the table below.

Commonly Used Theophylline Preparations

Form	mg/ml	Comment	Duration
Liquid			
Accurbron	10	—	6 hours
Elixophyllin	5	—	6 hours
Slo-Phyllin	5	no alcohol	6 hours
Somophyllin	18	no alcohol	6 hours
Fast-release tablets			
Slo-Phyllin	100,200	scored	6 hours
Slow-release beads			
Slo-bid Gyrocaps	50,100,200,300	capsule	12 hours
Theo-Dur Sprinkle	50,75,125,200	capsule	12 hours
Somophyllin-CRT	50,100,250	capsule	12 hours
Slow-release tablets			
Theo-Dur tablet	100,200,300	scored	12 hours
Quibron T/SR	300	scored	12 hours

Almost all our patients use the slow-release preparations. Even infants can use these bead preparations. The capsules can be opened and the beads poured into a spoon of applesauce, sherbet, jelly, peanut butter, or whipped cream. Chewing causes early release of the theophylline. After mixing, the beads should be swallowed immediately to prevent them from dissolving since this can cause early release of theophylline into the bloodstream. Fast swallowing also prevents the bad taste which occurs when the beads dissolve. Don't give theophylline beads in a baby bottle because it is impossible to judge whether the whole dose was taken. Many children aged eight and over can swallow theophylline tablets without difficulty. They must be swallowed whole or split as indicated. At the beginning of an episode, rapid and slow-release theophylline can be taken together to reach an effective level more quickly. However, since this frequently causes vomiting, most parents prefer to use an inhaled adrenergic drug along with slow-release theophylline to achieve the same effect.

Time Factors: Liquid preparations reach a peak level in the blood in one hour. In most cases they must be taken every six hours to maintain this level. Rapid-release theophylline tablets produce a fully effective blood level in about two hours and in most cases must be taken every six hours to maintain this level.

Slow-release preparations, Slo-bid Gyrocaps, Theo-Dur tablets, Theo-Dur Sprinkles, Somophyllin-CRT capsules, and Quibron T/SR tablets are usually taken every twelve hours. They begin to work within an hour and usually produce an effective blood level about two to six hours after the second dose, that is, in fourteen to eighteen hours. Once-a-day theophylline preparations are not

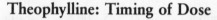

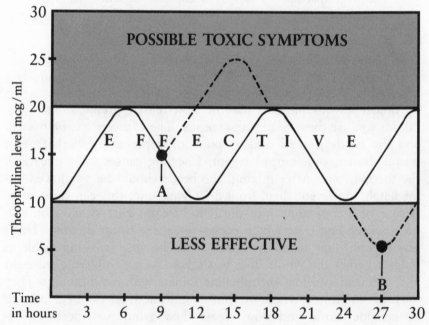

In this idealized graph, a slow-release theophylline preparation produces a serum level between ten and twenty mcg/milliliter if taken at twelve hour intervals. If taken three hours early (point A), it may produce toxic symptoms. If taken three hours late (point B), the amount of theophylline in the blood serum will drop to a less effective level.

recommended for children.

If the theophylline dose is taken too early, the amount of theophylline in the blood may reach toxic levels and adverse effects may appear. If a preparation is taken too late, asthma symptoms may reappear.

How to Give: Theophylline preparations should be taken at regular intervals to ensure that the serum level is both effective and safe. Though a deviation from the schedule of an hour or two often does not cause a problem, it is a good idea to establish a set routine.

Each theophylline preparation has its own advantages and disadvantages. These include absorption characteristics, ease of administration, dosage forms, dose amount, degree of stomach irritation and effect of food on absorption. For this reason most doctors limit themselves to one or two brands which they learn to use well.

Dosage: Doses are individualized but a common starting dose is 16 mg/kg/day or 400 mg per day, whichever is lower. The dose can be increased by twenty-five percent every three days until the desired effect or a toxic level is reached. Once an effective dose is established, it can be started immediately for subsequent episodes. Younger children metabolize (break down) theophylline more rapidly and thus need to take more theophylline per pound to achieve the same blood level as older children and adults. The table below lists dosages which usually produce the desired effect without causing toxicity. A blood theophylline level should be drawn if adverse effects (see p. 80) are prominent or increasing. A safe and effective blood level usually lies between 10 and 20 micrograms (mcg) per milliliter. A level should be drawn before exceeding the daily dose listed below to make sure that it is not in the toxic range.

Daily Theophylline Dose

Infants	calculation based on age and weight	
1–8 years	24 mg/kg/day	11 mg/lb/day
9–12 years	20 mg/kg/day	9 mg/lb/day
13–16 years	18 mg/kg/day	8 mg/lb/day
17 and over	13 mg/kg/day	6 mg/lb/day

Obtain blood theophylline level before exceeding this dose

The dose calculations should be based on ideal body weight. This means that an obese child will need less medication than a thin child of the same weight. Children under one year of age often break down theophylline more slowly than other children and usually require a dose ranging from 8 to 24 mg/kg/day. Their blood levels should be followed more closely than those of older children.

Many children will attain relief of symptoms and normal peak flow rates at doses lower than those listed above. This is particularly true if a child takes another drug at the same time as theophylline. In this case there is no reason to push the theophylline dose higher.

Some children eliminate theophylline from the body faster than average and will need to take a higher dose than usual. They may

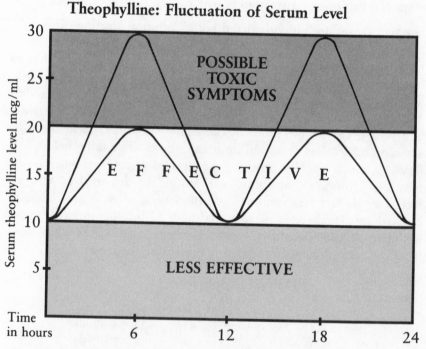

Theophylline: Fluctuation of Serum Level

Theophylline Serum Level: Only theophylline preparations which cause a fluctuation of less than one hundred percent from trough to peak serum levels are both effective and safe. Two out of twenty-nine brands studied in 1986 (Hendeles, p. 251) met these criteria.

also need to take it more frequently, for example, every eight hours instead of every twelve. Viral illnesses, including upper respiratory infections, fever, and some drugs (for example, erythromycin and oral contraceptives) may slow the elimination of theophylline from the body and reduce the amount needed. Smoking cigarettes or marijuana, eating charcoal broiled food or taking the drug phenytoin (Dilantin) may lower the theophylline level.

To insure that treatment will be both effective and safe, the physician should choose a theophylline preparation in which the highest (peak) blood level does not vary greatly from the lowest level (trough). A variation greater than one hundred percent is not acceptable.

A 1986 article (Hendeles) reported that of seven bead-filled capsules sold under sixteen brand names only one preparation, Slo-bid Gyrocaps, fluctuated less than one hundred percent from trough to peak. Eight tablet preparations sold under eleven brand names were also studied. Only Theo-Dur tablets produced serum theophylline concentrations within the acceptable range. Half of the bead-filled capsule preparations and half of the slow-release tablets had a peak-to-trough fluctuation which would exceed one hundred fifty percent in the average child.

Steroids (Corticosteroids)

■

THOMAS F. PLAUT, M.D. AND EMLEN H. JONES, M.D.

Steroids are extremely valuable drugs in the treatment of asthma. Occasional short-term use does not cause significant adverse effects. Between ten and twenty percent of our patients have required short-term treatment with steroids at least once over the past year.

Desired effects (These are all unique to steroids):

- to decrease swelling of the bronchiole lining by blocking movement of cells to the inflamed area.
- to reduce production of mucus by cells lining the bronchioles.
- to decrease hyper-reactivity of the airway.

- to restore responsiveness of airway smooth muscle to adrenergic drugs.
- to prevent formation of substances called leukotrienes which cause bronchoconstriction.

Generic names of short-acting steroids include prednisone, prednisolone and methylprednisolone. There are many brands. Generic preparations are safe, effective, and inexpensive.

SHORT TERM USE OF ORAL STEROIDS

Indications:

- Moderate or severe episode which does not improve significantly using an inhaled adrenergic drug.
- Episode which occurs in a patient who is already taking maximum doses of theophylline and/or an adrenergic drug.
- Mild to moderate symptoms which persist after several days of aggressive bronchodilator treatment in the absence of sinus infection.

Adverse effects: Adverse effects of corticosteroids are related to the quantity, frequency, duration, and timing of the dose given. They are most often seen when steroids are given on a daily basis for more than two weeks. Treatment for less than two weeks may cause an increased appetite, a feeling of well-being, fluid retention, and weight gain. The good feeling may be followed by moodiness when the steroid is stopped. Stomach upset, sometimes caused by steroids, can be reduced by giving them with food.

Form:

- Liquid
- Tablet

Time factors: Some effect is seen in three to six hours. It reaches its peak by twelve hours and lasts for thirty to thirty-six hours.

Dosage: Prednisone dosage is 1 to 2 mg per kilogram (about 0.5 to 1.0 mg per pound) up to a maximum of 60 mg per day for short term use. Steroids are often given one or two times a day for three to seven days in an acute flare. This short steroid burst can be discontinued abruptly without tapering the dose. In fact, tapering increases the risk of adverse effects by prolonging exposure to the drug (Iafrate, 1986). After stopping steroids, children over the age of four should be followed by peak flow meter readings to insure that their condition remains stable. Younger children should be observed closely for the return of symptoms and signs of asthma. If steroid treatment is required for more than fourteen days, gradual reduction (tapering) of the dose is advisable.

INHALED STEROIDS

Selected Steroids for Inhaled Use

Generic Names	Brand Names
beclomethasone	Beclovent, Vanceril
triamcinolone	Azmacort
flunisolide	Aerobid

Indications:

- child whose symptoms cannot be controlled after a fair trial of a combination of adrenergic drugs, theophylline, cromolyn, environmental control, and/or allergy injection treatment.
- any child who requires short-term oral steroid treatment more than six times within six months may benefit from treatment with inhaled steroids.

Dosage: Usual dose is one to four puffs taken two to four times a day. This varies with the drug used and the patient's age and condition.

Comments: Many patients can use inhaled steroids for long-term treatment. Using this inhaled route, the medicine is delivered directly to the bronchioles; small doses are thus effective. These small doses have not been shown to cause significant adverse effects. Inhaled steroids must be taken on a daily basis to be effective. It often takes one to four weeks for inhaled steroids to exert their beneficial effect. Use of a holding chamber (see p. 112) increases deposition of steroid in the lung. This reduces the dose and cost of medication. The holding chamber also decreases the deposition of steroid in the mouth making a yeast infection of the mouth unlikely (Toogood, 1984). Inhaled steroids are of no help in the treatment of an acute asthma episode, but should be continued during an episode to maintain their effect.

LONG-TERM USE OF ORAL STEROIDS

Oral steroids are the last medications used for long-term maintenance. However, steroid treatment can enable a child with severe asthma to lead a normal life. Duration of use may vary from four weeks to more than a year. Serious side effects may occur with careless or prolonged use. Long-term adverse affects can be avoided or greatly reduced by giving steroids in a single dose every other day at about 8:00 A.M. The body's natural steroid production is high in the early morning therefore this dosing schedule is less disruptive of the body's cycle. In our pediatric practice less than two percent of our asthma patients have used alternate day steroids for more than four consecutive weeks in the past year. A rare patient has required daily treatment for more than two weeks. Allergists and pulmonologists who care for patients with more severe asthma problems use steroids more frequently. They agree that long-term oral steroids should be used only when other treatment programs have failed to enable the child to lead a fully active life.

Indications:

- child whose symptoms cannot be controlled after a fair trial of a combination of adrenergic drugs, theophylline, inhaled steroids, cromolyn, environmental control, and/or allergy injection treatment.
- any child who requires short-term oral steroid treatment more than six times within six months may benefit from long-term steroid treatment.

Long-Term Adverse Effects (more than four weeks of daily use): Only a few of these changes may be noted at four weeks. The more significant changes come on gradually over a period of months. Steroids suppress the body's response to severe physical stress (major injury or surgery), inhibit linear growth, may cause cataract formation, acne, stretch marks on the skin, thinning of skin, increase in body hair, facial puffiness, headache, mood changes, high blood pressure, and loss of calcium from the bones which may lead to fractures.

Significant adverse effects are rarely seen with steroid treatment in a dose less than 30 mg every other day.

Form:

- Liquid
- Tablet

Dosage: The dosage for long-term use is adjusted to the individual patient's need and is usually much lower than standard short term dose. Most children do well on a single dose, between 5 and 20 mg, taken every other morning.

Who should not take oral steroids for more than two weeks? *

- the patient who has not worked out a written plan for asthma control with his or her doctor.
- the patient who has not tried various combinations of theophylline, cromolyn, adrenergic drugs and inhaled steroids administered by holding chamber or compressor-driven nebulizer.
- the patient with subtherapeutic theophylline levels who can increase the theophylline dose without inducing significant side effects.
- the patient with a sinus infection. Treatment of sinusitis will often lead to improvement of the asthma.

*Adapted from Guillermo Mendoza in *Asthma Update,* vol. 2, 1986 © David C. Jameson. Used with permission.

Cromolyn

Cromolyn taken prophylactically helps prevent the onset of asthma flares by blocking the release of chemicals which cause the asthma reaction. It is the safest drug used in the care of children with asthma. It is of no help in treating an episode which is underway.

Brand name: Intal

Indications:

- asthma which requires daily medication. Cromolyn helps about sixty-five to eighty percent of these children
- exercise-induced asthma
- episodic exposure to allergen such as animal dander

Desired effects:

- prevents release of chemicals from mast cells within the bronchioles which cause bronchospasm, swelling and increased mucus production
- reduces reflex-induced bronchoconstriction caused by cold air or exercise
- reduces bronchial hyperreactivity

Adverse effects: Cough, bad taste in mouth, and wheeze.

Form and Dosage:

- Starting dose, given four times a day, is the same for patients of all ages and may be cautiously reduced after one or two months of treatment. A full dose should be taken during the season in which the patient has the most difficulty. An occasional patient will regularly require a higher dose for full effect.

  Nebulized solution: Four ampules a day. This is the most effective route. A three-month-old child can inhale cromolyn by means of a compressor-driven nebulizer. It is often given simultaneously with an adrenergic drug.

Metered-dose inhaler: Four double puffs per day. Became available in the U.S. in 1986. Is easier to use and does not cause coughing as often as the inhaled powder does.

Powder-filled capsule: The powder from one capsule is inhaled four times a day using a special propeller inhaler (Spinhaler). More likely to cause coughing than the metered-dose inhaler or nebulized solution.

- After the first month the daily amount of cromolyn can often be taken in two doses, two to four puffs or one to two ampules each time.

Time factors:

- effective as a general preventative against asthma after one to four weeks of daily treatment.
- effective as a preventative against an allergen-induced episode if it is taken thirty minutes before exposure to the allergen (for example, cat or dog).
- effective as a preventative against exercise-induced asthma if taken a few minutes before exercise. Can be used following an adrenergic drug when neither cromolyn nor the adrenergic drug alone provides adequate protection.

Comments:

- The bronchioles need to be as open as possible for cromolyn to reach the small airways and become effective. A normal peak flow rate indicates that cromolyn will reach its target. A patient who has any symptoms of asthma must be treated aggressively and cleared before treatment with cromolyn is started or the treatment may fail.
- If the patient is under four years of age and thus too young for measuring the peak flow rate, some physicians give prednisone for the first week of cromolyn treatment to insure that the bronchioles are open.
- Some patients inhale an adrenergic drug before inhaling cromolyn to insure that the airways are open and prevent a cough during administration.

- Cough and bad taste in the mouth may be reduced by drinking a few sips of water before and after the inhalation.

- The occasional older child or teenager who cannot control a cough when inhaling cromolyn powder will usually tolerate cromolyn delivered by metered-dose inhaler or a compressor-driven nebulizer.

- Use of cromolyn may allow the patient to decrease or eliminate the daily theophylline dose in cases of perennial asthma.

- Cromolyn is not helpful in treating an asthma episode. However, its use should be continued during a episode unless it provokes significant coughing.

- The directions for use which are supplied in the package insert are clear.

Other Drugs

Combination Drugs: Most asthma experts now strongly oppose the use of more than a single drug in one syrup or tablet. In the past theophylline was often prescribed in combination with ephedrine (an adrenergic drug) and either a sedative or a tranquilizer. It is difficult enough to figure out how much of a single medication your child needs at a particular time. Rational treatment of asthma calls for the increase of a single medication to the point at which the patient either gets better or gets unacceptable adverse effects from the medication. Additional drugs are added as needed. With fixed drug combinations, one often gets adverse effects from one ingredient before getting full benefit from another.

Antibiotics: Are not helpful in treatment of an asthma flare unless there is a specific bacterial infection such as sinusitis.

Expectorants: Have not been shown to be effective in the treatment of asthma. Iodine preparations can interfere with the function of the thyroid gland.

Liquid: Drinking enough liquid (30 ounces for a thirty-pound child and 64 ounces for a ninety-pound child) will provide adequate hydration unless there is a fever or rapid breathing. Liquid intake should be increased by five percent for each degree of fever.

New Drug: Ipratropium (Atrovent) is a bronchodilator approved for use in the United States in the spring of 1987. It has been very helpful to a few of my patients who do not respond well to the usual treatments outlined in this chapter.

4

Home Treatment

Once you understand your child's asthma medications, you will begin to interact differently with your physician and your child. If your child's doctor prescribes a medication to be taken twice a day, you will ask whether the doctor means every twelve hours or twice a day as convenient. When your child begins to wheeze with exercise, you will realize that your current medication program is inadequate or that he or she needs pre-treatment before exercise. If your child's symptoms return three hours after using an inhaled medication, you will know that there is a problem somewhere: poor technique, worsening asthma, or inadequate dose. In each case the situation calls for review and remedial action.

As you gain knowledge you will notice that your physician, who had difficulty communicating with you last month, is now making more sense. Your physician will be more likely to pay attention to your observations and appreciate the questions you ask. He or she will consider your suggestions for a change in timing or dose of medication more seriously once they are based on knowledge rather than guesswork or hearsay.

Your doctor will probably not agree with every detail of treatment outlined in this book. That is fine. Our own treatment programs have changed each year for the past ten years and will change again next year. There are many ways to treat asthma. Whether your physician prefers to use an oral rather than an inhaled preparation of an adrenergic drug, or a fast-release rather than a slow-release theophylline preparation, is not important. The main requirement is that the entire routine fits together in a logical fashion, allows your child to have full activity, and allows you to lead a sane life.

When we see a new patient with an acute asthma episode, we prescribe a standard routine of treatment and then follow the child's progress closely, in the office or by phone, making changes as his or her condition requires. The parent keeps a detailed asthma record (see page 68) and comes back a week later—the next day in the case of a severe flare—to review the episode and talk about making adjustments for the next one. By the third episode, we have usually worked out an effective plan that the parent can handle independently. We ask the parent to keep records of each episode so we can continue to refine the treatment plan. We also ask the parent not to make changes in the plan without consulting us in advance.

Only in the mildest cases are we able to work out an effective treatment plan in a single visit. Sometimes several months elapse before the parent and the pediatrician have established the right medications, the right route of administration, the right dose, and the proper dosing schedule. The major decisions are made based on our knowledge of the patient, the severity of his or her asthma, and the family's circumstances. A four year old with moderate asthma who goes to day-care may require a program different from that of a similar child who is at home, and has the full attention of a parent or baby-sitter.

Mild asthma can often be well-treated with a single drug. For example, the child who gets a tight chest when running may be relieved of symptoms by pre-treatment with an inhaled adrenergic drug. The child who has a cough as the only symptom of asthma will usually benefit from treatment with a slow-release theophylline preparation. The young child with a mild wheeze may be treated with slow-release theophylline or an oral adrenergic drug. Usually the dose of these medications can be increased if symptoms do not clear completely with the starting dose.

Do not abandon a drug because you don't get the desired effect when you first use it. Some parents have told me their child gets no benefit from using an adrenergic drug by inhaler. In many instances, however, after the child learned proper inhaler technique or began to use a holding chamber (see p. 112), the medication produced good relief. Many of my patients find the hyperactivity induced by theophylline troublesome. Often I can eliminate the problem by giving the same amount in three rather than two doses per day. Sometimes lowering the dose of theophylline and adding an inhaled adrenergic drug produces the best result in terms of bronchodilation, convenience and avoidance of adverse effects.

Do not make any change in medication without the approval of your doctor. The parents of some patients have confided in me that they would rather lie to their doctor than have the doctor scold them for not giving medication as prescribed. In my opinion there is no room for scolding and no room for lying in the treatment of asthma. If you provide inaccurate information and your doctor changes the medication plan based on this information, your child may suffer. If you and your doctor cannot agree on a routine for the home treatment of asthma it is time for you to find a new doctor (see How to Choose a Doctor, p. 203).

You have the knowledge, but not yet the skill, to handle an asthma episode at home if your answers to all the questions in the Asthma Quiz at the end of this chapter are correct.

The Peak Flow Rate

Asthma usually does not attack without warning. An asthma episode is gradual in onset and also gradual in resolution. Thus, warning signals may be difficult to detect. Early changes in the small airways cannot be felt by the untrained patient or detected by standard means of physical examination. Usually when the patient feels tightness in the chest or starts to wheeze, he or she is already far into the episode. A doctor or parent can detect wheezing with a stethoscope, but only after the child's airways have been narrowed significantly. Treatment should be started before this point is reached.

Many children do not perceive any symptoms until a great number of their airways have been blocked. Often they will ignore symptoms as long as possible. The child with an asthma flare may find taking a deep breath uncomfortable and take shallow breaths instead. Since wheezing is more noticeable during deep breathing, the child unknowingly eliminates the wheeze.

The job of parents is to learn to identify the more subtle early warning signals of asthma. Once the importance of these warning signs is clear to parents, they will be able to treat an asthma episode much earlier and more effectively. The most reliable early warning sign of asthma is a drop in the child's ability to breathe out quickly, called the peak expiratory flow rate. By the time a physician or parent can detect wheezing with a stethoscope, the peak flow rate has dropped twenty-five percent or more.

Several new and inexpensive breathing monitors, known as peak flow meters, have proved useful for managing asthma in the doctor's office and the patient's home. Almost any child, four years of age or older, can learn to use one of these devices. They are durable, reliable and easy to use. Standard models can be used by both children and adults. We often recommend a low-range model for children under eight years of age because it has a smaller mouthpiece and an expanded scale.

Low Range Mini-Wright Peak Flow Meter

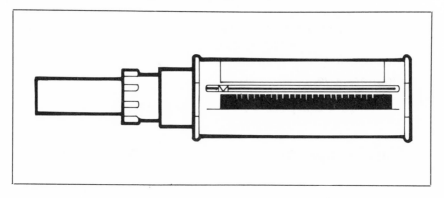

Measuring the peak flow rate in the office helps us to:
- diagnose asthma
- diagnose exercise-induced asthma
- monitor the patient's progress as we treat a flare in the office
- demonstrate the benefit of an inhaler

- demonstrate to a parent that the child needs to take more medicine
- distinguish between asthma and hyperventilation

Who should use a peak flow meter? Most children age four and over will benefit from using a peak flow meter at home to show that they are doing okay and do not need to start or change medication. A twenty percent drop from the child's "personal best" peak flow rate indicates the need to increase the medication dose or frequency. An increase after taking medicine is clear evidence that the medicine was needed.

With the meter, a parent can check to make sure that the child's condition does not worsen when medication is reduced. If the peak flow rate remains stable, the parent can reduce medication further with less risk of a relapse.

A parent can also use the meter to predict an asthma episode. Often, the peak flow rate will often drop twenty-four hours before the symptoms of an attack are noticeable. This early warning allows some parents to start giving medication early.

A drop in peak flow may indicate that it is time to look for triggers of asthma in the environment. Finally, a drop in flow should prompt you to look for the early clues of asthma (see p. 53). You will find that the peak flow meter is a valuable tool in learning about and monitoring your child's asthma.

Peak Flow: The Key to Asthma Treatment

The peak flow meter is the key to success in asthma treatment. Much more sensitive than the stethoscope, it is the most useful device available to monitor asthma treatment at home. Every asthmatic child over four years of age should learn how to use this instrument.

The peak flow rate varies over a twenty-four hour period. It is highest between noon and 6:00 P.M. and lowest between midnight and 6:00 A.M. Intervention should begin early if the peak flow rate begins to drop during the day. An abnormally low morning reading also identifies an undesirable state. Your child may require treatment, even if the peak flow rate improves spontaneously during the day, if the rate of improvement is slow.

Most parents get acquainted with the peak flow meter by checking their child's rate three times a day. This should be done before an inhaled adrenergic drug is taken. After a few weeks parents reduce or discontinue formal monitoring of peak flow measurements unless their child is in trouble or continues to have low peak flow readings. The asthma record (see p. 68) provides space for recording peak flow rates.

Assess Peak Flow Monitor

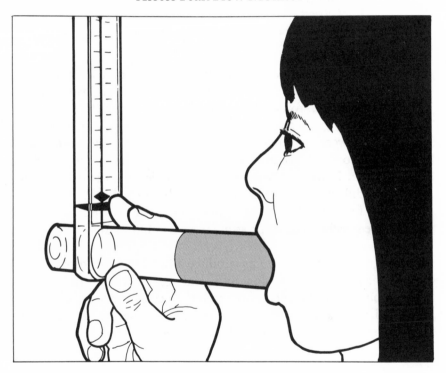

To use the peak flow meter your child should:

1. Remove gum or food from mouth, and move the pointer to zero.
2. Stand up, and hold meter horizontally with fingers away from vent holes and the marker.

3. Slowly breathe in as much air as possible with the mouth wide open.
4. Put the mouthpiece on the tongue and place the lips around the mouthpiece.
5. Blow out as hard and fast as possible—a short sharp blast. The meter measures the fastest huff, not the longest. Therefore, ask your child to give a fast blast, not a slow blow.
6. Huff three times, waiting at least ten seconds between huffs and moving the pointer to zero after each huff.
7. Record the best huff morning, noon, and night. Try to do this at the same time every day while learning about asthma or during an asthma flare.

Note: If a peak flow attempt causes your child to cough, this usually means that his or her asthma is not adequately treated.

What is a normal score (maximum peak expiratory flow rate) for your child? The huff is related to height in children and is measured in liters per minute. You can get a rough idea of your child's normal value by checking the chart below. However, there is a great deal of difference between children. The best way to find your child's normal value is to check the huff several times when he or she is feeling perfectly fine. Consider the highest value achieved on two occasions to be your child's "personal best." This is the normal value and reference point for your child until it increases. An increase may be due to improved technique, improvement in asthma status, or normal growth.

Problems with technique can produce a falsely low reading. These include inadequate effort, slow huff, leakage of air from the corners of the mouth or a blockage of the mouthpiece by the tongue. We are interested in measuring the child's maximum capacity to huff. For this reason we *never* average peak flow attempts.

Guidelines for Peak Flow Rate

Peak flow rates vary somewhat by sex and race. In a study of the peak flow rates of three ethnic groups, white and Mexican-American males showed average rates about fifteen percent higher than black males (Hsu, 1979, see p. 252). The average rates for females were ten percent lower in each of the three ethnic groups. These differences are small compared to the changes that take place in an individual during an asthma episode.

Peak Flow Rates in Liters per Minute

Height in inches	Average rate	Range*	Height in inches	Average rate	Range*
40	150	110–190	56	330	240–420
41	160	115–205	57	340	245–435
42	170	120–220	58	360	260–460
43	180	130–230	59	375	270–480
44	190	135–245	60	390	280–500
45	200	145–255	61	400	290–510
46	210	150–270	62	415	300–530
47	220	160–280	63	430	310–550
48	230	165–295	64	445	320–570
49	240	175–305	65	460	330–590
50	250	180–320	66	480	345–615
51	260	190–330	67	500	360–640
52	270	195–345	68	515	370–660
53	280	200–360	69	530	380–680
54	300	215–385	70	550	395–705
55	315	225–405	71	570	410–730

*includes 95% of white males age seven to twenty years.

Derived and adapted from Katherine H. K. Hsu, Daniel E. Jenkins, Bartholomew P. Hsi, Erwin Bourhofer, Virginia Thompson, Frank C. F. Hsu, and Susan C. Jacob. 1979. Ventilatory Functions of Normal Children and Young Adults—Mexican-American, White, and Black. *Journal of Pediatrics.* 95:192–96.

Each child has his or her own pattern or type of asthma episode. Most episodes come on gradually and a drop in peak flow rate can alert the parent to start medication before actual symptoms appear. This early treatment can prevent a flare from getting out of hand. Occasionally episodes come on very quickly. The peak flow meter can confirm their onset and eliminate some of the guesswork in treatment.

Mini-Wright Peak Flow Meter

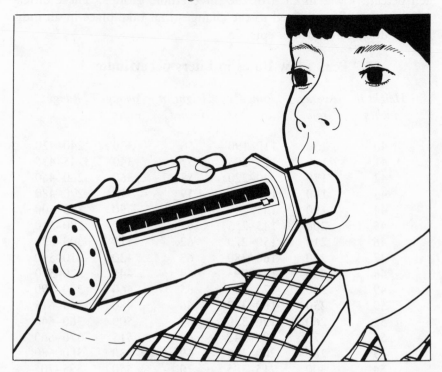

Peak Flow Zones

Best Huff	100	200	300	400	500	600
Green						
80–100%	80–100	160–200	240–300	320–400	400–500	480–600
Yellow						
50–80%	50–80	100–160	150–240	200–320	250–400	300–480
Red						
0–50%	0–50	0–100	0–150	0–200	0–250	0–300

Home monitoring may be done morning, midday and evening (roughly 7:00 A.M., noon, 7:00 P.M.). It can easily be done at school. If your child takes an inhaled drug, measure the peak flow rate before treatment and five to ten minutes after. One way to look at peak flow scores is to match three zones of peak flow with the colors of the traffic light. Green (80–100 percent of personal best) means all clear: hold at present routine or reduce medication. Yellow (50–80 percent of personal best) means caution: an increase in medication may be needed. Red (below 50 percent of personal best) calls for a full evaluation with your doctor.

For example, if a child's best huff when he or she is feeling fine is 300, her green zone would be above 240, yellow 150–240, and red less than 150. The peak flow for a child increases with improvement in asthma. We record the best blast of three attempts as a measure of the childs maximum capacity to breathe out. Do not average several attempts. Peak flow measurements are like the high jump. You get three tries and the best one counts. One or two low huffs out of three tries are almost always due to poor technique. In a child who knows how to huff, three low huffs indicate a real problem.

The available standards for mean peak flow based on height are useful only as an initial guide to peak flow. For example, if a patient blows 400 when the mean peak flow for height is 350, the 400 should be used as the standard for that patient until he or she exhales (blasts out) at a higher rate on two occasions. A high figure produced by a cough or a whip of the neck does not count.

The following guidelines for treatment based on peak flow are general in nature. You should discuss them with your physician and adjust them to fit your child's needs. Your plan may differ from this one.

The green or O.K. zone: In this zone, the child has full breathing reserve and no symptoms. A mild trigger may not cause symptoms. For example, a mild upper respiratory infection, jogging, or cold air may well be tolerated in this zone. If asthma symptoms occur, usually they come on slowly giving adequate notice to begin treatment.

If your child's peak flow, before you give medication, is in the green zone regularly for a forty-eight-hour period, you may consider

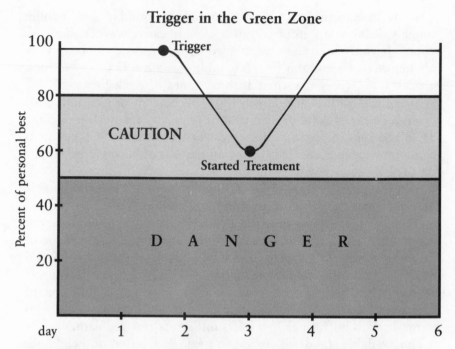

This child's peak flow rate is 95 percent of his personal best. An upper respiratory infection triggered an asthma episode and his breathing reserve dropped to 60 percent. He noted a slight wheeze, started to take medicine and recovered quickly.

reducing the dosage of medicine or reducing the frequency of administration of medicine according to a plan worked out in advance with your pediatrician.

The yellow or caution zone: The child has reduced reserve, and may have mild or moderate symptoms. A minor trigger produces noticeable symptoms. A combination of several triggers, for example, exposure to cigarette smoke combined with an upper respiratory infection, may produce significant breathing trouble. Two peak flow scores in the yellow zone within forty-eight hours usually indicates that you should add to the present treatment. A child operating with a peak flow at seventy-five percent of personal best may have no symptoms while he is in a quiet clean environment. However, if he laughs, jogs, or goes outside in the cold, he may cough, wheeze or complain of a tight chest. He is living in the yellow zone. Though his difficulties are not obvious to him or his parents, he is vulnerable to asthma triggers. They may bring on symptoms so quickly that

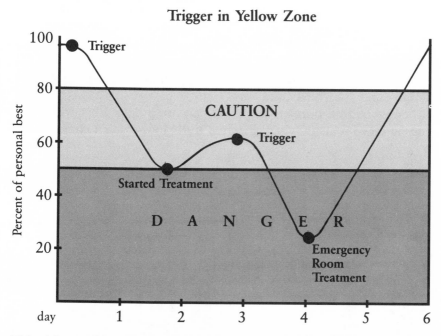

Trigger in Yellow Zone

This girl started having symptoms after she developed an upper respiratory infection. Her wheezing improved with medication, but after thirty-six hours was still present at rest and she was not feeling well. Her peak flow was 60 percent of her "personal best." When she encountered an additional trigger she started having severe difficulty and required emergency room treatment.

they cannot be controlled effectively by usual treatment. It may take several days of treatment before his symptoms disappear completely.

Red, danger or doctor zone: If your child's peak flow is in the red zone (before treatment) twice within a forty-eight hour period there is a definite problem. You should review this situation in the office with your physician. If your child can not give a good effort for the peak flow test, his or her rate is probably in the red zone.

Why should you give asthma medicine to your child if he or she has no symptoms? The purpose is to maintain a good reserve breathing capacity so they will not get into trouble quickly when they confront a trigger.

Asthma can be better managed by determining daily peak flow levels at home than by obtaining full pulmonary function studies once a month in the doctor's office (Williams, 1982). Since the peak flow rate is the most sensitive measure of lung function available for home use, its results should be taken seriously. However, using the peak flow meter is not a substitute for understanding how your asthma and your medicines work.

Some children thirty months old can use a peak flow whistle. It can be set to whistle when the child huffs in the green zone.

Peak Flow Monitor

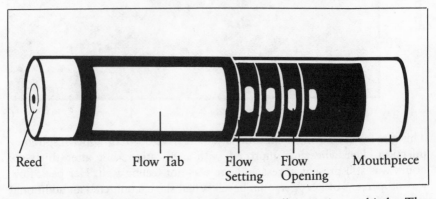

Reed   Flow Tab   Flow   Flow   Mouthpiece
                                     Setting   Opening

Air flowing through the reed at a certain rate will cause it to whistle. The rate of airflow depends on the patient's peak flow and also the number of flow holes opened in the peak flow monitor.

Two types of patients have been found to run into serious trouble with asthma. One type procrastinates, accommodating to symptoms such as a cough and wheeze. When they encounter a trigger they have little or no breathing reserve and will get into trouble quickly.

The other type overreacts to symptoms and often takes more medicine than is necessary. The peak flow meter can help parents of each type of patient learn when to start, adjust, and stop medications.

Some physicians say that the peak flow meter is too technical for use at home. They say that learning about this aspect of asthma care is too demanding and may make a family overinvolved with asthma. We believe that they are like physicians who think that checking urine or blood sugar levels at home is too complicated for the family of a diabetic child. These doctors have no idea how much fear, anxiety, and disruption uncontrolled asthma causes in a family. Certainly there is a lot to learn. However, parents of our patients are willing to learn if it will improve their child's health.

Comparison of Peak Flow Meters[a]

	Mini-Wright	Low range Mini-Wright	Assess	Peak Flow Monitor
Age (years)[b]	6 and up	4 to 8	7 and up	$2^1/_2$ and up
Reliability	excellent	excellent	excellent	excellent
Ease of Reading	excellent	excellent	good	good
Ease of Use	excellent	excellent	excellent	good[c]
Approx. Cost	$29.95	$35.95	$19.95	$12.95

[a]For ordering information, see vendors in resource list.

[b]Based on peak flow rates for height. See table on p. 101.

[c]Set at 80 percent of personal best. Whistle indicates effort is in the green zone. Easy to use at a single fixed setting. Somewhat cumbersome to move flow tab.

Timing of Treatment

An asthma episode develops gradually and is often due to multiple triggers. The obstruction often increases over a period of days rather than a period of hours. Recovery usually takes equally long. Most parents start treatment too late and stop it too early. They should start treatment when they first notice an early clue or the first symptom of an asthma problem: a night cough, cough with exercise, or the first tiny wheeze. However, many parents do not give medication at the onset of wheezing but rather wait to see what will happen. In our practice we say, "Wishing won't work," and "Hoping won't

Timing of Treatment

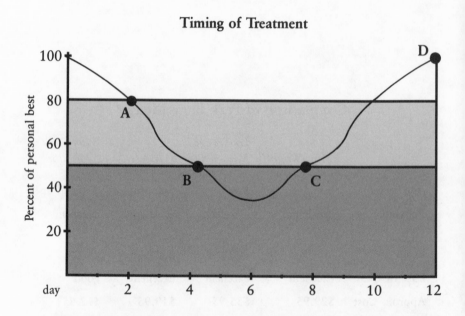

You should start treatment when peak flow drops into the yellow zone (A). Many parents wait until symptoms are very noticeable; upon entering the red zone (B). At this point swelling and increased mucus production may cause symptoms to worsen despite treatment with bronchodilators. Parents often discontinue medication when symptoms improve (C) instead of tapering after child's peak flow scores have been in the green zone for forty-eight hours (D). Adapted from A. Bergner and R. Bergner, "Does Asthma Attack?" Unpublished paper. Used with permission.

help." Asthma medicine should be started at the first hint of an asthma problem and continued for at least two days after all signs of the problem have disappeared. Stopping medication prematurely leaves the child vulnerable to worse breathing trouble if the original trigger is still present or another trigger appears in his or her environment. In children over the age of four, the peak flow rate can often define the onset of a flare a day or two before symptoms are evident. It can also define when recovery is complete.

Parents and doctors often talk about the relapse of asthma symptoms as if the initial problem had been completely cleared. "Relapses" often occur because an asthma flare has been only partially treated, either with an inadequate drug program or for too short a time.

Inhalation Devices

We prescribe inhaled adrenergic drugs for three-quarters of the more than four hundred children with asthma in our practice. Children ages three to ten often have great difficulty timing inhalation to match delivery of the mist from the inhaler. The bad taste of the medication accentuates this problem. Children ten or older also may have trouble with timing. For this reason we usually recommend some device to aid in the delivery of inhaled adrenergic drugs. It is difficult or impossible for infants and young children to use a metered-dose inhaler (MDI) properly.

There are two groups of devices that parents and children can use to assist in the administration of inhaled medications. The compressor-driven nebulizer is recommended for children under three years of age and any other child with asthma who has difficulty using the MDI or a holding chamber. This includes children who usually do well with these devices but have too much difficulty breathing to use them effectively in the middle of an episode.

COMPRESSOR-DRIVEN NEBULIZER

The parents of young patients say the compressor-driven nebulizer is a godsend. These machines have been used to treat asthma in

Compressor-Driven Nebulizer

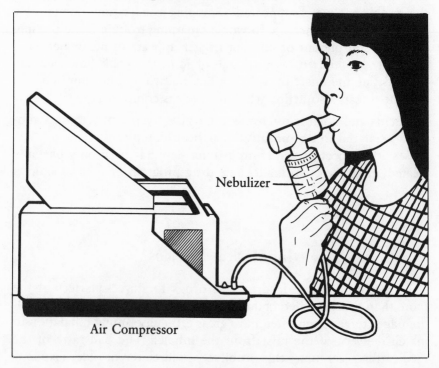

hospital wards and emergency rooms for many years. We believe that
unless office staffing or space is inadequate, children with moderately severe asthma should usually be treated with adrenergic drugs
by compressor-driven nebulizer instead of with painful adrenalin
shots. The medication mist travels right to the bronchioles. Thus less
medicine is needed and adverse effects are minimized.

The compressor-driven nebulizer, also known as the air compressor nebulizer, works by forcing air past a solution that contains medicine, producing a fine mist. The child inhales this mist through a
mouthpiece or a mask while breathing normally, or if possible, holds
his or her breath for a second at the end of each inhalation.

In our office the nurse instructs the parent as she measures out the
medicine, places it into the nebulizer unit and gives treatment.
Thirty minutes later the parent takes over the job for a second treat-

ment. If the child has improved satisfactorily the parent goes home with a compressor-driven nebulizer and the medication needed to treat the episode.

Use of the compressor-driven nebulizer has enabled parents to care for their young children at home instead of subjecting them to the trauma of emergency room treatment or a hospitalization. Even if hospitalization becomes necessary, a compressor-driven nebulizer can reduce the length of stay. Since children can continue treatment at home with a compressor-driven nebulizer, they don't have to wait for complete clearing before discharge.

Aside from its use in preventing and shortening hospital stays, the compressor-driven nebulizer enables parents to administer cromolyn to children under age four. Heather and Nathan in chapter one used cromolyn by compressor-driven nebulizer.

Who should consider buying a compressor-driven nebulizer? First, anyone whose child has been admitted to the hospital or treated in the emergency room more than once. Second, anyone whose child would benefit from cromolyn therapy and cannot inhale cromolyn by another method.

Prerequisites for Use of Compressor-Driven Nebulizer at Home

The physician should be clear that the parent:

- knows the four signs of asthma trouble
- uses a peak flow meter if the child is over age four
- understands fully the child's medication
- is willing to keep an asthma record
- has been trained in the use and care of the compressor-driven nebulizer
- has a written plan for its use

The compressor and attachments cost between $130 and $260 for the same machine depending on the dealer. It is worth checking for the best price. If instruction is not given by the physician's staff, there may be an additional charge for setup and instruction by a respiratory therapist. Two of the most commonly used compressors, Medi-Mist (Mountain Medical Equipment, Inc.) and Pulmo-Aide (Devilbiss Company) should be available from local distributors. If not, you can contact the company directly for purchase information (see p. 248). A prescription is required. Enough albuterol or meta-proterenol for thirty treatments costs about $10.

Many doctors have told me that they felt compressors were too expensive for their patients. In fact, the opposite is true—many families cannot afford to be without one. These machines prevent emergency visits to the hospital and to the doctor's office. Since these visits usually cost between $66 and $200, the compressor pays for itself in one or two visits. To top it off, many insurance plans will pay eighty percent of the cost.

HOLDING CHAMBERS

All holding chambers catch the mist from a metered-dose inhaler and hold it until the child starts to breathe in. This eliminates the need for perfect coordination between release of the mist and inspiration. It allows the mist to be breathed in at a slower, more effective rate (Levison, 1985). In large-volume holding chambers, air dilutes the unpleasant taste of medication, making it easier to breathe in. Adverse medication effects are reduced because the large particles of medication are often trapped in the chamber before reaching the mouth.

InspirEase

We call this collapsible large-volume reservoir "the accordion" because it makes a musical sound if the patient breathes in too fast. Since slow inhalation leads to greater deposition of the medication mist in the bronchioles the sound is a very helpful feedback feature. The InspirEase is collapsible and easy to carry. This is the best holding chamber I have seen for children ages five and over. Younger children may have difficulty breathing in slowly and holding their breath for five seconds. It costs about $12 from Key Pharmaceuticals (see p. 249) and requires a prescription.

InspirEase Holding Chamber

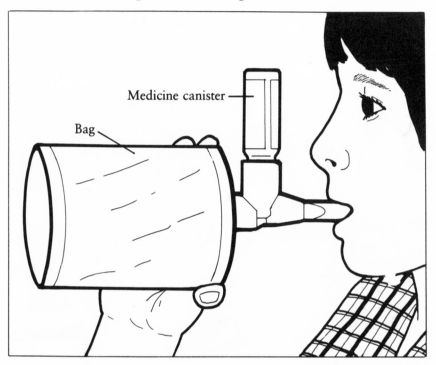

Medicine canister

Bag

Instructions:

1. Extend bag.
2. Place the mouthpiece on your tongue and puff one whiff of medication into the chamber.
3. Suck in slowly with lips snug around mouthpiece and hold breath five seconds.
4. Breathe out, keeping lips snug around mouthpiece.
5. Suck in slowly and hold breath five seconds.
6. Repeat full procedure with a new dose of medication after waiting at least two minutes.

INHAL-AID Holding Chamber

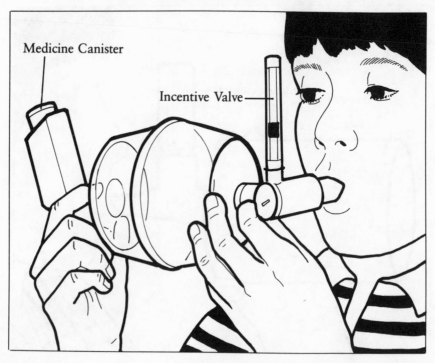

Medicine Canister

Incentive Valve

Inhal-Aid

Most three-year-olds can use this large-volume device with a metered-dose inhaler (MDI) after a few practice sessions. A special feature is the incentive marker which indicates adequate inspiration. The INHAL-AID can be used with good effect in a mild or moderate episode. An ability to hold the breath is not required. This is a very effective holding chamber for children ages three to six. It costs about $15–20 from Key Pharmaceuticals (see p. 249) and requires a prescription.

Instructions:

1. Place mouthpiece on tongue.
2. Puff one whiff of medication in the chamber.
3. Suck in with lips snug around mouthpiece and hold breath for five seconds.
4. Continue to hold lips snug around mouthpiece and breathe out.
5. Suck in, hold breath, and breathe out three more times.
6. Wait at least two minutes and repeat the entire procedure with a new dose of medication.

For Younger Children Who Cannot Hold Their Breath:

1. Place mouthpiece on tongue with lips snug around mouthpiece.
2. Puff one whiff of medicine into chamber.
3. Encourage child to inhale, raising the float to the top, if possible, ten times in a row; the slower and higher the better. Some children get good results with less than perfect technique.
4. Wait at least two minutes and then repeat the whole routine if prescribed.

Paper Tube

Children over six who have difficulty coordinating the release of medication from a MDI with their inhalation will find a paper tube holding chamber helpful.

Instructions:

1. Roll a piece of typing paper to form a tube eight inches long and two inches in diameter.
2. Puff one whiff of medication in, then inhale with lips snug around the tube.
3. You must start to inhale slowly within one second and hold your breath for five to ten seconds.
4. Repeat routine after waiting at least two minutes.

Paper Tube Holding Chamber

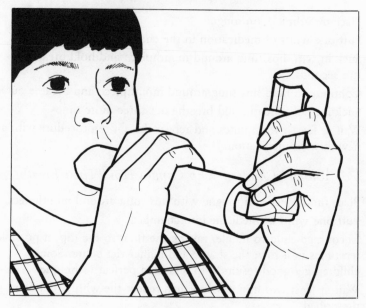

Aerochamber Holding Chamber

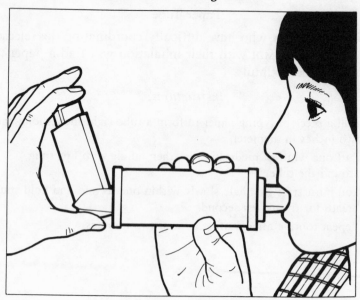

AeroChamber

This commercial version of the small-volume holding chamber has a valve which prevents accidental exhalation of the medication. For best effect, the inhalation must be held for ten seconds. Repeat routine after waiting at least two minutes. It costs about $12–$14 from Monaghan Medical Corporation (see p. 249), and requires a prescription.

Comparison of Holding Chambers

	InspirEase	INHAL-AID	AeroChamber	Paper tube
Volume	700 cc	700 cc	150 cc	150 cc
Feedback Effort	Yes	Yes	No	No
Feedback Flow	Yes	No	No	No
Portability	Good	Fair	Good	Good
I recommend for Age in Years*	5	3	6	6
Price	$12	$15–20	$12–14	$0.01

* Some well-coordinated children can use at an earlier age.

Large-volume chamber dilutes medication taste more effectively. Flow feedback feature trains the patient to draw air in slowly. This maximizes deposition of medication in the bronchioles. Effort feedback feature lets the patient and parent know that the child is breathing in and making a good effort.

Medication Routines

The four common medicines available for the prevention and treatment of asthma can be used in various combinations. Parents and patients have a choice of several different medication routines. Different families will make different choices even though their asthma problems may be the same. Their decision takes into account the child's age, chronicity of asthma, triggers of asthma, rapidity with which episodes come on, severity of flare, usual duration of episode, significance of adverse effects, ease of administration (frequency, timing, mechanics), and cost.

For intermittent asthma (occasional asthma symptoms which do not require long-term treatment on a daily basis), the choices of medication are adrenergic drug by inhalation, adrenergic drug by mouth, theophylline, and prednisone.

Inhaled adrenergic drugs have the benefit of being effective within minutes. Since only a small dose of the drug is used, adverse effects are usually not significant. The disadvantages are that they require proper technique, the effect lasts only four to six hours, and inhalation devices are bulky. Minor shakiness is a common adverse effect.

Adrenergic drugs by mouth (liquid or tablet) are sometimes recommended for children who have been shown to have fewer side effects from an adrenergic drug than theophylline. They are easy to give. The disadvantages are that the effect lasts only six to eight hours. Since the dose is much greater than for the inhaled adrenergic it is more likely to cause shakiness.

Theophylline is usually prescribed as a long-acting preparation and is effective for eight to twelve hours. It is convenient both to take and to carry. Common side effects are hyperactivity, stomach ache, and headache.

Prednisone is never used alone but rather as a second or third drug in combination with an adrenergic drug and theophylline. It is often used in the case of a severe episode; if a trial of an adrenergic drug and theophylline has not brought adequate improvement over a specified time, or if previous episodes progressed rapidly despite aggressive treatment with bronchodilators.

In order to avoid emergency room visits and hospitalization, you and your physician must work out a treatment routine that is aggressive and is based on the usual pattern of your child's asthma. Pay close attention to the duration of action of the various drugs. Recurrence of symptoms before the next dose of medicine is due means that the medication program is not adequate. The routines given here have worked for our patients; however, many other possibilities exist.

STARTING MEDICATION

Inhaled adrenergic drug chosen as initial drug: At the first sign of an asthma episode the patient takes one treatment of an inhaled drug. One treatment is defined as any one of the following:

- two whiffs of the metered-dose inhaler, with at least a two minute interval between the first and the second.
- one puff into a holding chamber using INHAL-AID, InspirEase, AeroChamber, or a paper tube, then repeat two minutes later.
- a single compressor-driven nebulizer treatment.

If this provides significant relief within less than fifteen minutes and there is no regression of symptoms over the next four hours, the patient can continue to use this treatment alone, that is, one treatment every four to six hours while awake—and also if awakened during the night. If symptoms recur before four hours pass, the treatment is inadequate and the patient must start taking theophylline (make sure you have it on hand). Improvement should occur within two to six hours after the second dose of theophylline. Call your physician for advice if the child gets worse or the expected improvement does not occur. In this situation you will usually be asked to come to the office for a check.

Theophylline chosen as the initial drug: You should see significant improvement within two hours after giving the second dose of theophylline. *Your child's condition should not worsen while you are waiting for theophylline to reach its full effect.* If your child's condition does get worse at any point or you don't see significant clearing within two hours after the second dose of theophylline, add an inhaled adrenergic drug. If symptoms don't clear in fifteen minutes after taking the adrenergic drug or if they recur in the next four hours, an office visit is probably necessary.

Two-drug treatment (adrenergic drug plus theophylline): If your child has a history of developing a severe attack in a short period of time that does not respond to a single drug, it makes no sense to repeat a plan that has failed in the past. In this case, we recommend use of two drugs as soon as symptoms are noted.

Prednisone: For severe attacks that don't respond to an adrenergic drug plus theophylline, we often recommend a short burst (three to seven days) of prednisone. Some of our patients with a history of severe episodes have a limited amount of this medication at home. A rare child will require prednisone and an inhaled adrenergic drug at the beginning of an attack. This determination is made on the basis of previous experience and/or present examination findings.

The parents of every child who has been admitted to the hospital or has required emergency treatment for asthma should be taught to use at least two drugs by their physician. These drugs should be kept at home, packed for every vacation, and available for use without further consultation with a physician.

STOPPING MEDICATION

During the first asthma episode, since neither we nor the parents know the pattern the episode will take, we arbitrarily recommend giving medication on a regular basis for a full week. We usually reexamine the patient at this point to see that his or her peak flow is normal and to review the course of the episode. We reduce medication gradually after the patient has been free of all asthma symptoms (cough, wheeze, rapid breathing, wheezing with exercise) for two days.

One learns about asthma with each episode by keeping a proper asthma record. The medication routine should be modified to fit the child's usual pattern of symptoms and response to treatment. The rest of this discussion refers to subsequent episodes.

Inhaled adrenergic drug: After your child has been without symptoms or signs of asthma for two days, omit one of the daily treatments, spacing the remainder equally over twenty-four hours. For example, if you were giving four a day, reduce them to three. If the symptoms and signs of asthma do not return, continue to drop one treatment per day. If symptoms recur it is wise to increase the frequency of administration immediately.

Long-acting theophylline: After your child has been without symptoms or the four signs of asthma trouble for two full days, give one-half the dose for twenty-four hours. If symptoms do not recur, discontinue theophylline. Once twenty-four hours have passed without symptoms, further medication is not usually needed. If symptoms reappear it is wise to restart theophylline at full dosage right away.

Two-drug routine: If your child is using an adrenergic drug as the primary drug, discontinue theophylline in two steps as described above. If no symptoms recur within twenty-four hours after the last dose of theophylline, follow the single-drug routine for the adrenergic drug.

If your child is using theophylline as a primary drug, discontinue the adrenergic drug as described above. If no symptoms recur in the twenty-four hours after the last adrenergic dose, give one-half the usual dose of theophylline for twenty-four hours. Continue as in the theophylline routine above.

Three-drug routine: If your child is taking an adrenergic drug, theophylline, and prednisone, the prednisone is discontinued first, usually after three to seven days, provided the patient has been asymptomatic for at least two days. If no symptoms recur in the forty-eight hours after the last dose of prednisone was given, discontinue the second and third drugs, as described above.

Remember, you cannot wish an asthma episode away. Treatment must be aggressive, based on the pattern of your child's episodes and on the duration of action of the various medicines used. For children four years old and over, you can use peak flow rates as a guide to starting and stopping medications.

For patients who have chronic asthma which requires daily medication for more than a month at a time, the same principles of medication practice hold. The additions and subtractions are just made to an existing medication base of theophylline, cromolyn, or inhaled steroids.

Instructions for Treating an Asthma Episode

Instructions for the management of an asthma episode are too complicated simply to be given orally. There are many opportunities for errors by the physician, the pharmacist, and the parents. Medicine with a single name may come in several strengths and dosage forms. Often a child must take several medications simultaneously.

The form below allows the physician to provide individualized directions for the parent in an efficient manner. It also gives a parent the opportunity to look at the instructions and ask questions about them in the office. Last but not least, it eliminates the need for guesswork in recall after leaving the office. Some general comments follow.

- You and I will modify your child's medication routine as we gain more experience in treating his or her asthma.
- Asthma episodes are usually triggered by exercise, viral respiratory infection, cigarette smoke, allergens and cold air.
- Avoid cigarette smoke and the smoke from wood burning stoves.
- Stay away from cats and dogs if there is any indication (sneezing, itching, wheezing or coughing) that an allergy exists.
- Use acetaminophen instead of aspirin if aspirin has been shown to trigger an attack as it does in two percent of children with asthma.
- Your child should drink a normal amount of liquid each day for his or her size. This is about one quart for a thirty-pound child and two quarts for a ninety-pound child.
- High fever or rapid breathing increases the body's need for liquid.
- Continue taking cromolyn or inhaled steroid during an episode unless it causes coughing.
- Please check the previous chapter for adverse effects of each medication.
- Do not buy a new allergy-causing pet such as a cat or dog if your child is being treated for asthma. It makes sense to dispose of an animal if your child is allergic to it.

Medication Instructions

____ Give inhaled adrenergic drug as
_____, one treatment by inhaler,
holding chamber, or nebulizer every four hours the first day
and then up to four times in twenty-four hours until there
are no symptoms and peak flow is normal for two full days.
Reduce by one treatment a day if symptoms do not recur
and peak flow is normal.

____ Give theophylline _____ mg per day as
_____ _____ mg every _____
hours. After there are no symptoms and the peak flow is
normal for two full days, reduce the dose by fifty percent. If
symptoms do not recur in the next twenty-four hours stop
theophylline.

____ Start both inhaled adrenergic drug and theophylline at the
above dose. After your child has had no symptoms and the
peak flow is normal for two days, taper one drug and then
the other as outlined above.

____ Give adrenergic drug by mouth, as albuterol, metaproterenol
or terbutaline _____ mg per day as _____ mg or _____ cc
every _____ hours.

____ Give prednisone or prednisolone _____ mg per day as _____
mg at the following times _____
for _____ days. Give as _____ 5, 10, or 20 mg tablets or
_____ cc liquid at each dose.

**Do Not Reduce the Theophylline Dose or Reduce the Adrenergic
Dose to Less Than Three Times a Day Until 48 Hours *AFTER
COMPLETING* Steroid Burst.**

____ If worsening at any time or not greatly improved after four
hours of treatment, call the office.

____ Call the office if you have any questions or think the doctor
or pharmacist has made an error.

Asthma Quiz

Accurate knowledge of the basic facts about asthma and the medications used to treat it are essential if parents want to communicate fully with their child's doctor. It also provides the foundation they need in order to take on a significant part of the responsibility for managing their child's asthma at home.

1. What are the four signs of asthma trouble?

    1. _____   3. _____

    2. _____   4. _____

2. Name three changes in the bronchioles caused by asthma.

    1. _____

    2. _____

    3. _____

3. Name one early clue that your child shows before he or she

    starts an asthma episode. _____

4. Name one event which triggers an asthma episode in your child.

    _____

5. Why should you give medication to prevent an asthma episode?

    _____

6. Why should you give medication early to treat an episode?

    _____

7. How long should your child take medicine for an asthma episode? _____

8. How much liquid should your child drink in twenty-four hours with an asthma episode? _____

9. Under what circumstances should the blood theophylline level be checked? _____

10. Answer true or false. When using adrenergic inhaler:

   a. Breathe in as deeply as possible _____

   b. Hold the breath for ten seconds _____

   c. Always take a double whiff, unless doctor says otherwise _____

   d. Allow two-minute intervals between whiffs _____

   e. Inhaler can prevent wheezing set off by exercise _____

   f. More effective if used when standing up because then one can take a deeper breath _____

   g. Clean plastic case with warm soapy water, then rinse once a week and when there is dirt or film on the tiny exit hole _____

11. What medication does your child take?

Name	Strength in mg.	Action	Time to Reach Full Effect	How Long Effect Lasts

ASTHMA QUIZ: ANSWERS

1. (a) Wheezing; (b) chest skin sucked in; (c) breathing out takes longer; (d) breathing rate changes

2. (a) Muscles around the bronchioles tighten up; (b) lining of the bronchioles swells; (c) mucus is produced by cells inside bronchiole.

3. Cough, sneeze, watery eyes, tight chest, gets upset, other

4. Infection, exercise, cigarette smoke, allergen, cold air, laughing.

5. It is easier to prevent an episode than to treat it. Before an attack the three responses in the bronchioles haven't started.

6. Medication works better before swelling and mucus become severe. It takes only minutes to relax tight bronchiolar muscles but days to clear up swelling and mucus.

7. Until all symptoms have disappeared and peak flow is normal for two days, unless your doctor says otherwise. See Medication Routines.

8. A thirty-pound child should drink about one quart; a ninety-pound child should drink about two quarts of liquid.

9. (a) If there are any concerns about theophylline toxicity;
   (b) before increasing the dose above the usual for age.

10. All true.

11. This is a selected, representative, not an all-inclusive list:

Name	Strength in mg.	Action*	Time to Reach Full Effect	Effect Lasts
Theo-Dur tablets	100,200,300	1	two to six hours after second dose is given	12 hrs
Theo-Dur sprinkles	50,75,125,200	1		12 hrs
Slo-bid	50,100,200,300	1		12 hrs
Quibron T/SR	300 (3 score)	1		12 hrs
Slo-Phyllin	60,125,250	1		8 hrs
theophylline tablet	100,200,300	1	2 hr	6 hrs
theophylline liquid	varies	1	1 hr	6 hrs
adrenergic liquid	10,20	1	30 min	6 hrs
adrenergic inhaled	varies	1,5	30–60 min	4 hrs
prednisone tablet	5,10,20	2,3	12 hrs	36 hrs
prednisone liquid	5 per 5 ml	2,3	12 hrs	36 hrs
prednisolone liquid	5, 15 per 5 ml	2,3	12 hrs	36 hrs
cromolyn	0.8,20	4	1–4 wks	days
		5	15 min	4 hrs

1. Dilates bronchioles, 2. Reduces swelling. 3. Reduces mucus production
4. Stabilizes mast cells in airways. 5. Prevents exercise-induced asthma

5
Families and Asthma

Asthma is like an unwelcome visitor. You didn't ask for it, but since it's here, you'd better learn to deal with it. If you don't, asthma will intrude in all aspects of your family's life. Asthma can be kept under control once you get to know it and become assertive in your dealings with it.

When you first begin learning to manage an asthma episode at home, most of the activity is under the control of your child's doctor. After you and the doctor have worked out a plan to manage an episode, you will gain confidence. Soon you will be able to manage most episodes at home, using what you have learned from your doctor, your reading, your discussions, and your own experiences.

One of the first benefits of knowing how to keep a flare from getting worse is the conviction that you are in charge, not the asthma. Educated parents can give better care because they know when to seek help. They can judge when home treatment is working and when to see the doctor.

Putting parents in charge of controlling their child's asthma does not mean that the doctor is abandoning the patient. In the best of situations, parents will be dealing with a physician who will assure them that she or a substitute will be available at noon on Christmas Day or midnight on July the Fourth as well as during regular office hours if they should need a phone consultation.

In our pediatric practice, we invite parents to education sessions to learn about asthma and to meet other parents who are managing their children's asthma at home. In other places, parents have taken the initiative to form their own support groups. In Pittsfield, Massachusetts, the American Lung Association responded to a mother who wanted to form a support group and continues to provide staff assistance to the parents' group. In New York City, a support group was born in a hospital pediatric intensive care unit when two mothers introduced themselves.

Helping Parents Manage Asthma

Knowledge of asthma and the medicines used to treat it is essential if you want to manage your child's asthma at home. But knowledge isn't enough. Parents need to develop the skill to make accurate observations of their child's breathing, to interpret peak flow readings and to use holding chambers and compressor-driven nebulizers. After attaining these skills, they must develop an attitude that allows them to try these new behaviors. Many parents are frightened of an asthma episode, afraid that their child may die if not rushed to the doctor immediately. Our parents' education/support group has changed parents' attitudes in a dramatic way.

Nine years ago, I started the group with the help of Sharon Dorfman, a health educator. The goals of the program are:

- to increase parents' knowledge of facts and myths about asthma, its treatment and the prevention of episodes.
- to provide a comfortable setting for sharing feelings about the ways in which asthma affects the child, parents, and others.
- to build the family's skills in monitoring the child with asthma, recognizing the onset of episodes and making appropriate decisions about using medications, contacting doctors, and dealing with schools, friends, and babysitters.

A great deal of information is presented at the first session. Much of it has been covered with parents during office visits. However, reviewing this material with twelve to sixteen parents who are at various stages of learning about asthma is a great help. This is the first time that some parents see that others are dealing with the same problems as those they are struggling with day-to-day. In the second session we use a sentence completion exercise to bring out prevailing attitudes of fear, anger, guilt and pessimism that exist in the parents of children with a chronic illness. Once in the open, these feelings can be discussed and related to by all parents.

We work to create a positive attitude by demonstrating that parents can manage various practical problems. Parents learn from each other how to cope with overnight visits, problems with teachers, dealing with doctors, and the fright of an acute episode. This learning among parents helps them feel less dependent on the doctor and more ready to handle problems on their own.

Once parents have acquired the knowledge and skill to handle an episode, and have gone through some attitudinal changes, they are able to behave in an effective manner. They can treat a flare early, will know how to judge progress, and will be able to control asthma rather than letting it control them.

Optimal management is only possible when the parent gets support and guidance from the physician consultant. We ask the parent to bring the child to the office at any time if they are unsure of their ability to judge the severity of an episode. At the visit, we compare the parents' observations and assessment with ours. In that way, they can increase their knowledge and skill in dealing with asthma at each visit. We are available for consultation twenty-four hours a day on every day of the year if a child with asthma has a serious problem. This means that our parents don't have to worry that their child will be cared for by an unknown physician in an unfamiliar way. With this kind of support, parents have learned to become confident managers of their children's asthma.

Parents' Asthma Group

During four hours crammed with information, demonstrations, practice, and discussion, parents have an opportunity to consolidate their knowledge of asthma and its treatment. They discuss their feelings with parents who have had similar experiences. They find that their reactions to asthma and to the disruptions it causes in their lives are shared by many others. The group gives them a chance to get better acquainted, in a relaxed atmosphere, with the physicians who will take care of their children when they are having trouble.

After parents have participated in the asthma group, they become more capable of monitoring their child's asthma and of handling episodes. Their increased knowledge and skills result in a more confident attitude and less of a tendency to restrict the child. The children increase their participation in sports and social interactions. The family as a whole functions better because the stress on it is reduced.

Some of these changes are illustrated by comments obtained from several mothers three months after they attended the initial parents' asthma group sessions in 1978.

> . . . feel more secure about treatment. I can now call in when Matt has an attack and change dose by phone with my physician's help, based on the report I give him.
>
> . . . feel more secure about medication, and not worried about giving Mike an overdose and killing him. I feel more confident about when he should be seen by physician. Asthma, itself, is unchanged.
>
> . . . found out Lindsay's problem is not as severe as we originally thought, compared to other children. I feel comfortable that my doctor has studied asthma and knows a lot about it. I feel that information before a crisis is worth its weight in gold. We are now able to anticipate and organize things.
>
> . . . much more comfortable with Josh's asthma. Recently he started wheezing at wilderness camp 100 miles away. The nurse called, frantic, at 7:00 A.M. and asked me to come and get him right away. I assessed the situation on the phone and gave instructions to the nurse for treatment. Josh remained at camp with his class. I was able to go to work.

Before parents attend our first education session, they receive printed information from our office. Between sessions, they are asked to fill out a questionnaire about how they, their children, and others feel about the child's asthma. After each session they are asked to fill out an evaluation sheet.

Parents' Asthma Group: Initial Information

Goals: To increase parents' knowledge of the facts and myths about asthma, its treatment, and the prevention of asthma attacks. To provide a comfortable setting for sharing feelings about the way in which asthma affects the child, the parents, and others.

To build the family's skills in monitoring the child with asthma, recognizing the onset of flares and making appropriate decisions about environmental control, using medications, contacting practitioners, and dealing with schools, friends, and babysitters.

Who is invited: Parents of children with asthma who are patients at Amherst Medical Center.

When and where: Two two-hour sessions one week apart. Both sessions will be held in the obstetrics waiting room at Amherst Medical Center. Individual consultations will be provided at the end of each session.

Since the second session builds on the learning and sharing of the first, only parents who attend the first meeting may participate in the second.

Preparation: We are counting on everyone to read Chapters 2, 3, and 4 of *Children With Asthma: A Manual For Parents* before the first session so that we can have more time for discussion.

Fee: $40.00 per family for the series. Those in the Health Plan are already covered.

Staff: Drs. Thomas F. Plaut and Emlen H. Jones (second session).

For more information: Call the pediatric office and ask for one of the nursing staff.

Complete and return the enclosed registration form and the asthma visit questionnaire if you wish to attend.

Parents' Asthma Group: Registration Form

If you decide to participate in the group, please complete this form and send it to Pediatrics. Your thoughtful responses will help us plan a program that reflects the backgrounds, concerns and interests of group members.

How interested are you in learning about the following?

Please rate on a scale of 0 to 5. (0 means "not at all", 5 means "strongly interested")

_____ asthma medications

_____ asthma and sports

_____ breathing exercises

_____ controlling the environment of a child with asthma

_____ early clues that an episode may soon start

_____ how asthma is diagnosed

_____ the effect of asthma on overall health

_____ the relationship to allergies

_____ the role of emotions

_____ things that may trigger an episode

_____ what happens in the body during an episode

_____ when to seek medical assistance

_____ others (please list) _____

Please feel free to add any other questions, interests or areas of concern related to asthma that you would like to suggest for inclusion in the series.

Name of Child: _____

Parents' Names: _____

_____

Phone Numbers: (Home) _____

(Work) _____

By registering early, you reserve a place in the next Parents' Asthma Group. Once the dates are set, we will contact you to confirm. At that time you will be asked to make a commitment to attend both sessions.

Agenda for First Session of Parents' Asthma Group

7:30 Get acquainted: Give your name, the name and age of your child, duration of his/her asthma, an asthma concern; and make an unrelated comment.

7:40 Introduction: We have these sessions to help parents understand asthma so they can see that their child gets the proper treatment when he/she needs it.

7:50 Breathing: Chest and lung structure and function.

8:00 Asthma attack: Constriction of smooth muscle, swelling of windpipe lining, secretion of mucus.

8:10 Triggers: Infection, exercise, irritants, allergens and mechanical. Indirect (weather and emotions).

8:20 Early clues: Important in deciding when to medicate.

8:30 Five minute stretch.

8:35 Keeping records: Helps in adjusting medication amount and duration.

8:45 Severity: Parents can judge it accurately, using wheezing, retraction, in-out ratio, and breathing rate.

8:55 Medications: The two main drug types are adrenergic drugs and theophylline.

9:10 Questions

9:25 Evaluation sheet: Need evaluation sheet to plan next session.

9:30 Individual consultations.

Please fill out the feelings sheet and fill out an asthma record for the week before the next meeting.

Feelings: Parents' Asthma Group

Please complete these sentences before coming to the second session.

1. I think that having asthma makes my child feel

2. Because of asthma, I think others treat my child differently by

3. When my child has an asthma attack, I wish I was able to

4. I feel angry when

5. Because of asthma, I treat my child differently by

6. The aspect of my child's having asthma that frightens me most is

7. I feel guilty about

8. During an asthma attack, I become frightened when

9. When dealing with children who have asthma and their parents, I wish that doctors would

10. When an asthma attack occurs, I think my child feels

11. My child's reaction makes me feel

Agenda for Second Session of Parents' Asthma Group

7:30 Environmental factors: Pollutants include cigarette smoke, wood stoves, paint, perfume.

7:40 Allergic factors: Triggers include animal dander, pollen, and house dust. Which child needs allergy evaluation?

7:50 Feelings: Discussion will focus on the sentence completion exercise.

8:20 Prognosis: How serious is asthma? Does anyone outgrow it?

8:25 Five minute stretch.

8:30 Other medications: Steroids, cromolyn.

8:40 Peak flow meter: Its use at home to guide treatment.

8:45 Inhalation devices: Compressor-driven nebulizer and holding chambers.

8:55 Instructions for parents. Information for school nurse, teacher, and emergency room doctor.

9:00 Questions.

9:25 Evaluation.
Set date for three month's follow-up meeting.

9:30 Individual consultations.

Evaluation Sheet: Parents' Asthma Group

Date: _____

Before you leave, please share with us your honest reactions to tonight's session on this anonymous form. Your thoughtful responses will help us improve future sessions.

1. What are your feelings about the:

	Excellent	Satisfactory	Less than Satisfactory
Clarity of information presented	———	———	———
Comfort created for participation	———	———	———
Leader's ability to hold interest	———	———	———
Leaders' receptivity to questions, ideas, and comments	———	———	———
Leaders' sensitivity to group members' concerns	———	———	———
Organization of session	———	———	———
Quality of sharing in the group	———	———	———
Relevance of content to you	———	———	———
Usefulness of the session to you	———	———	———
Overall evaluation	———	———	———

Comments:

Which topics needed *more* time?

Which topics needed *less* time?

2. Please circle your opinion about:

Amount of information	too much	too little	about right
Level of information	too basic	about right	too technical
Length of session	about right	too long	too brief

Pace of session	too fast	too slow	about right
Group size	too small	about right	too large
Opportunities for group sharing	about right	too many	too few

3. Did you:

Learn new information?	a lot	a fair amount	a little
Change any perceptions?	a few	not really	many
Share your concerns/ideas with the group?	a lot	a little	a fair amount

4. What did you learn or relearn that will help you most in dealing with asthma?

5. What could have been done differently to improve the session?

Other comments and suggestions are welcomed. Thank you.

Stages in Parents' Ability to Manage Asthma

No Knowledge: Cannot recognize an asthma episode. Knows nothing about medicines.

Beginner: Can recognize an asthma episode. Needs help in deciding when to start medicine. Cannot judge severity of attack. Cannot communicate clearly with physician on phone.

Intermediate: Can handle an episode well with doctor's help. Knows how to judge severity of a flare, how to use a peak flow meter and when to start treatment. Can communicate clearly with physician by phone giving description of progress.

Advanced: Has good knowledge of early clues, triggers and medicines. Skilled in monitoring an episode and use of medicines. Can handle most episodes at home without consulting physician. Has instituted some environmental controls.

Expert: Excellent knowledge, skill, and attitude. Can handle almost all episodes without consulting physician. Has instituted reasonable

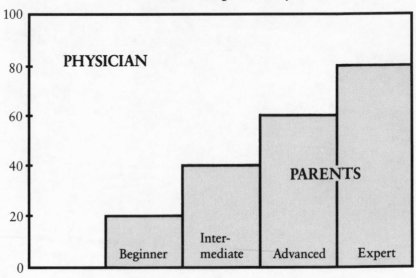

Shared Responsibility

environmental controls. Understands the usual course and patterns of child's episodes. Able to analyze episodes and make suggestions to physician that improve treatment. Still needs physician for special situations and integration of new medications and treatment at three- to twelve-month intervals.

Parents should share the responsibility of managing a flare with their physician. You should learn something from every office visit and every asthma episode. The best tool for learning about asthma is the asthma record. Write your observations and peak flow readings on it and you will be able to analyze the effects of various triggers and medications.

Feelings

An asthma episode is always inconvenient and often disruptive. If you don't know how to take care of it, the episode can be very frightening, too. When your child has trouble breathing and you don't know what to do, you become anxious, excited and scared. Your distress has an unsettling effect on your child. The only thing you can think of is to get help as fast as possible.

Your child misses school. You have to miss work, in order to care for him or take him to the doctor. You feel that you are not in control of events. You have less energy to spend on other members of the family. Plans are disrupted. You have to cancel or cut short family outings. Your child misses a basketball game or has to cancel an overnight visit.

Asthma is nobody's fault. You get angry that it happened to your family. There is nothing fair about asthma, arthritis, diabetes, or a seizure disorder. Its occurrence is beyond a family's control. However, the outcome of an asthma episode usually can be significantly affected by the family's knowledge, skill, and attitude in managing the problem.

During the first session of the parents' asthma group, parents receive basic information about asthma and the medications used to treat it. At the end of that two-hour session, they are given a "Feelings Sheet" to fill out at home (see p. 136). This gives them the opportunity to think about the new information and their attitude toward asthma and its effects on them and their child. By the time they get together for the second session of the parents' asthma group, parents realize they have a lot in common. A great deal of discussion takes place during the sentence completion exercise on feelings.

In a group of twelve parents, several will come up with the same words and phrases when asked how they, the child and others feel about the child's asthma.

Asked how the asthma makes their children feel about themselves, common answers are:

- Like most other kids.
- Haven't noticed a difference.
- Different.
- Different from other kids and often angry.
- Frustrated that he cannot do everything he'd like to.
- Frightened, anxious, tired.
- Cautious.

Between episodes some children are able to ignore their asthma completely. Other children have to be alert to triggers and early warning signs of an episode. This helps them to prevent some episodes and treat others early. A few children have asthma that is so severe that despite good management skills they get into difficulty.

Parents perceptions of how (or whether) others treat their children differently because of the asthma vary. Common answers are:

- They don't.
- Worrying about medicine time.
- Letting him take a break when he is playing sports. Otherwise, others don't treat him differently.
- Wondering how it affects her.
- Being overprotective.

It is hard to know how to deal with other people until you get your child's asthma straight in your own head. People who have a lot to do with your child—playmates, hockey coach, teacher, babysitter, friends' parents—should know enough about asthma to deal with it in a relaxed fashion without being overprotective or demanding too much when your child has an episode.

During an asthma attack, parents say they wish they were able to:
- Know why it's happening and judge the severity better.
- Help her relax and have a well thought-out plan of action.
- Feel sure about what I was doing right.
- Console him, encourage him.
- Breathe for him!
- Reverse it immediately.

Parents share many of the same angry feelings centering around children with asthma. They say they feel angry when:
- I have to miss a lot of sleep because of her asthma.
- An episode interferes with family activities for a prolonged duration.
- I sit here and feel that I'm dumb and don't know enough about what's going to happen.
- He won't help himself until the episode gets more severe.
- He does not take his medication and I know he needs it.
- He "uses" his allergies and asthma for attention or as an excuse.
- He forgets his medicine at a friend's house.
- I can't do anything to help him.

Asthma is not fair to parents. Sometimes you can do everything right yet an episode disrupts a family trip or forces you to leave work to care for your sick child. Asthma is not fair to children. They must be more responsible than their friends in monitoring their bodies and taking their medicines.

Do parents treat their children differently because of asthma, and if so, how? The most common answers are:
- I don't believe I do.
- Encouraging him to learn methods to cope with asthma.
- I don't, except to check how she feels before she starts something strenuous.

- Overprotecting sometimes, worrying about him more.
- Not letting him play as hard.
- Watching her too closely.

Most parents in the asthma groups know when they are being overprotective of their children. This is a usual early reaction in caring for a child with asthma. As you gain an understanding of asthma and your child's limits, you can shift from overprotection to sensible management.

Asked what aspect of their child's asthma frightens them most, parents answer:

- I don't feel frightened anymore; we understand how to handle it.
- There is none.
- She may not always be able to participate in any activity she wants.
- I won't know when or what to do.
- Possible ill effects of long-term medication.
- The possibility of not reversing a flare.
- That the breathing would become so difficult he'd not be able to.

Every parent whose child has severe asthma has worried about the child dying from an episode. Once they learn how to manage an episode, they worry much less. Actually, death from asthma is rare in childhood.

It is important to get feelings of guilt out into the open so that misplaced self-accusations can be looked at objectively. Asked what they feel guilty about, common answers are:

- I don't believe I do.
- Not knowing enough when she has an episode.
- Not detecting earliest signs.
- Getting angry when he's sick.
- The fact that the asthma comes from my side of the family.

In the past doctors thought asthma was caused by a defective mother-child relationship. We now know that there is no truth whatsoever in this theory. However, it is natural to feel some guilt when you have a sick child. Do not dwell on it but rather learn more about taking care of asthma and how to interact better with your child.

How does the child feel when an asthma flare occurs? Parents' answers to what they think their children feel include:

- Scared and angry that it's happening.
- Frustrated—"What, again?"
- Unhappy and sometimes frightened.
- Like sticking very close to mom and familiar surroundings.
- Sick, is what he says.

An asthma flare can be a scary, frustrating, disruptive, unhappy event. I never heard anyone say it was fun or even O.K.

The five things that parents mention most often when they are asked what frightens them during a flare are:

- The medication is not bringing it under control and her breathing becomes more labored.
- He coughs and can't keep his medicine down.
- She has to be hospitalized.
- He becomes gaunt, frightened.
- I think that I am losing control.

All of this is frightening and it is time to call for help.

One would think that a parent's answers would depend primarily on the severity of his or her child's asthma. Actually, two other factors are of equal importance: the age of the child and the ability of the parents to manage an episode. Under age four, children often get into difficulty quickly because their small bronchioles are blocked more easily. In addition, they are unable to use a peak flow meter. For both these reasons, parents are often unable to start asthma treatments early enough.

Parents who have the knowledge and skill to manage an episode go through their routine without becoming anxious. They start treatment early and vigorously. They can judge when treatment is effective and do not worry unnecessarily. They know when an episode is getting worse despite aggressive treatment and contact the doctor for help before things get out of hand.

Another group of parents is clearly heard from in these comments. They know that they could be in control of the situation, but for some reason—perhaps not enough experience, study or planning—they are not able to perform well enough to manage a standard episode. One mother said she almost wished her son would have another flare soon so she could improve her skill in managing asthma at home.

Finally, there is a group of parents who feel that they are not in control and don't see how they can be. Their presence in the parents' asthma group makes me believe that they will be able to learn to manage their child's asthma, as have hundreds of other families in our practice.

Support Groups

New support groups for parents of children with asthma are springing up at a growing pace. Since local resources and the orientation of parents vary greatly, each group is different.

Pittsfield Support Group

■

LYNN ARSENEAU

My daughter, Michelle, suffered for four years and had been hospitalized twice before I began to learn how to deal with asthma. Once I got her problem under control I felt the need to help others avoid what I had gone through.

Most parents are confused and helpless. We don't know the first thing about asthma or the medicines used to treat it. We treat our children like china dolls because we are afraid they may die with the next asthma episode. Many of us don't realize that our child's episodes can be prevented or brought under control. We don't know how much we can accomplish with the guidance of our own pediatrician.

We often experience feelings toward the child that are difficult to deal with. These feelings can create guilt and resentment. It's very important to discuss what we're feeling with people who are experiencing the same emotions. It's not the child we resent; it's the asthma. It's important to separate the child and the disease.

Before I started the support group, I contacted the American Lung Association (ALA) to find out if one already existed in my county. There was none. When I voiced my desire to begin a group, ALA offered to assist me. For the first meeting I invited a pediatrician who cares for many children with asthma. The ALA took care of contacting our local medical center to reserve a conference room. It also handled the publicity and direct mailings.

About fifty people attended. I started the meeting by telling a brief asthma story about my daughter and why I was starting a support group. The guest pediatrician explained the basics of asthma and then parents shared their own experiences and asked many questions. Judging from the questions during and after the meeting, it was very successful.

We have had several meetings since then. The ALA has been very helpful. It supplies us with handouts, coloring books, comic books about asthma, "Super Stuff" kits, "No Smoking" signs, booklets and more. It has handled all mailings, publicity, and room reservations. It has lent me films and a projector. Parents fill out evaluation sheets at the close of each meeting; this way we find out what worked and what didn't and also get suggestions for future meeting topics.

One Saturday afternoon I organized a program centered on the children. We played games that encourage effective breathing techniques. Each child talked about about his or her asthma and how it makes them feel. They also drew a picture of what they thought asthma looked like. We talked about what to do when they feel the "Big A" creeping up on them. They took home coloring books, buttons, "No Smoking" signs, pencils, and balloons. This meeting was my favorite. The best part was demonstrating what happens in the lungs during an asthma episode. We used balloons attached to the ends of straws as props.

Parents tell me that the group has really helped them in a number of ways. They now understand how medications work and what side effects they cause. Some now realize their child does not have a serious problem. A number of parents have learned to communicate better with their doctors. They are no longer afraid to ask questions or to present their points of view. Most of them now ask for written instructions when a new medication is prescribed.

The group helped one couple resolve a dispute about activity for their child. The mother wanted to limit activity because of asthma. The father thought that the child should have a normal schedule. The group discussed this, understood the mother's concerns, but felt that with adequate treatment full activity was in order.

I sometimes get phone calls at home from parents who need support during a difficult time. I tell them what has worked for me and for others. Since I'm not in the medical field I refer people to their doctors for medical advice. Though every child is different, the parents' problems often seem very similar.

New York City Support Group

■

PAUL JAEGER

This was our second "overnight" in the pediatric intensive care unit. Adam's asthma attack had not responded to three shots of epinephrine and the hospital recommended that he be admitted. The nurses got him all plugged up with needles and tubing and whatnot, including a cardiac monitor.

There was only one other child in the ward. Leonard was very young, and he too had tubing and wires spilling from his body. His parents, Cindy and Mark, had never been through this experience before. In fact they didn't even believe that their child had asthma, although he was under the care of a pediatric allergist.

My wife, Miki, went over to the other family, offering tea, a tuna sandwich, and a little sympathy. An asthma support group was born. With the help of our doctor we contacted a third parent whose child had asthma. Miki, Cindy, and Hannah talked on the phone often, getting help from each other—sharing their experiences and their fears. The children got sick, and they got better. Their mothers discussed new drugs, diets and nutrition, how the children got on with their peers, what to do when you are far from a hospital, and how asthma is misunderstood by most people.

The three families started getting together once a month, without the children, just to talk. We found other parents to join us, including our own doctor, an asthma specialist who has a child with asthma. We shared more of our fears, and our experiences. We invited guest speakers—experts in the fields of psychology, physical therapy, and pediatrics.

In every meeting we discuss, we argue, we laugh, and we cry. Every parent at the meeting gets a chance to tell not only how their child has been doing, but how they, themselves, have been doing. We hear how each individual copes with the emotional stress of their child's attacks, and how each deals with the medical questions as well. Cindy has told how she uses the inhaler whenever Leonard shows the first sign of an episode, and has not needed to go to the hospital for a long time. Sarah told of taking Joseph out of a hospital emergency room against medical advice and bringing him to another hospital, which was able to deal properly with his crisis. The group felt that Sarah did the right thing, both for Joseph's medical well-being and for their emotional health. Miki and I explain that we don't hesitate to increase Adam's medication at the slightest hint of a problem. We can make these decisions within certain guidelines worked out with our physician. The support and easy accessibility of the physicians who care for our children are important factors in building our competence and confidence.

Every parent has her or his own theories, and each of us has been willing to listen and learn from others as well as trying out our own ideas. As we learn more and more about asthma, we all have been able to take a degree of control over our child's medication and consequently our lives. Most of us have learned to sense an impending episode and administer the proper medications to halt its progress. Our doctors are happy that members of our group rarely find it necessary to call them in the middle of the night.

We share our successes. Cindy and Mark were going to cancel a summer vacation because of Leonard's asthma. With the support of the group and their new-found knowledge, they were able to go. Beth and John take Frank to Fire Island regularly. It is a long ferry ride to the nearest hospital but they feel secure, equipped with the supply of medicines which they take with them. Adam and I recently finished a 7000-mile tour of the Western United States, camping the entire way, usually many miles from the nearest medical facility. During the trip, Adam was exposed to untold dust and pollen. We had no trouble keeping his asthma under control.

Not long ago, a mother mentioned that her two-and-a-half-year-old daughter was afraid of the compressor-driven nebulizer and absolutely refused to use it. Another mother in the group volunteered to help solve the problem by having her three-year-old daughter demonstrate how she inhales the mist. The two mothers and their daughters got together for a morning of play. Halfway through, the three-year-old turned on her nebulizer and showed how she used it. Within a short time fear of the nebulizer was conquered.

Before we created the group, our children's allergies and asthma controlled many aspects of our lives. We couldn't go to Grandma's house because she had feather pillows. We couldn't take that trip to Europe for fear of an asthma flare over the Atlantic. And the circus was out because of all those hairy animals. We lived in fear of that next episode. We lived in terror that our child might literally die before our eyes. But knowledge of the disease and methods of controlling it now allow us to lead normal lives.

The group continues to grow. New parents—frightened, angry, denying their child's asthma—come to meetings where they find that we, too, have experienced those feelings and still feel them from time to time. The group has given strength to the individuals in it. The key has been a willingness to share our joys and our sorrows, our strengths and our fears, our insecurities as well as our knowledge.

Asthma is a Family Affair

In the vast majority of families, the mother takes on the major responsibility for managing a child's asthma. She is the one who administers the medication, she takes the child to the doctor's office, and she stays with the child when the child is hospitalized.

No matter who takes on the primary responsibility for asthma care, every member of the family is affected by this chronic illness. In a two-parent family, the father will get less time with his wife. He will often feel deprived of her company and resent his child's asthma. However, if he takes part and shares in the care of his child with asthma, the parents may be drawn closer together rather than separated by the illness.

Parents who are only minimally involved in the care of a child with asthma often do not have a clear understanding of what is going on. They may not understand the need for a visit to the doctor. They may be reluctant to spend money for medicine and equipment. They may become impatient when asthma care requires a lot of time and attention. On the other hand, sometimes the less involved parent overreacts, demanding that the spouse take the child to the doctor when the situation is actually under control.

If a father has had asthma as a child, he may remember that he had to "tough out" an asthma attack and expect his child to do the same. Of course, asthma treatment is much different today and "toughing it out" is no longer a sensible alternative.

A mother often will prefer to give asthma treatments with a compressor-driven nebulizer by herself because it's easier than teaching her husband. This may be true in the short run; it certainly is not in the long run. In the middle of a difficult episode, it is really helpful if a father can take over. Everybody needs to get some rest. It is not reasonable to expect a mother to work three shifts a day taking care of asthma. If a father takes over one night-time treatment from his wife, he will help to preserve her health and also establish a good connection with his sick child. His interest and involvement will help the family function better. His lack of involvement m~y pull it apart.

Some parents seem to be less patient than others. One wanted to smash the asthma equipment against the wall. Another wanted to flush all the medicine down the toilet. A third could not understand why there should be no smoking in the house. Once these parents learned about asthma, their patience with the treatment routines increased.

Brothers and sisters are also involved in asthma care. Older siblings often remind a child to take medicine and serve as advisors to inexperienced babysitters. They report symptoms to their parents and can also help younger siblings take an inhalation treatment or use a peak flow meter. One boy told his father not to smoke in the house because it caused trouble for his brother. Another read to his younger brother from the book, *Teaching Myself About Asthma.*

Grandparents are often very helpful as babysitters. They will sometimes take the kids when the parents go off for a weekend or a week's vacation. To make it possible for the grandparents to provide effective care, the parents should give them written instructions. They should teach the grandparents how to use all the devices that the child needs, (peak flow meter, compressor-driven nebulizer, and holding chamber). The grandparents should also know the four signs of asthma trouble, when to call for help, and how to interpret peak flow readings. Involved grandparents can often enjoy their grandchildren more because they feel comfortable about caring for a child with asthma. Other grandparents, who are less involved, often don't understand that certain aspects of their living conditions—for example, cigarette smoke or a favorite cat—can be a problem for the child with asthma. It is the parents' job to educate them. Grandparents are welcome to attend the Parents' Asthma Group.

In families of divorce, both parents should know about asthma and the medicines used to treat it. Each needs a written copy of the routines used in the management of their child's asthma. In our practice, divorced parents and their partners are invited to the Parents' Asthma Group. We do our best to communicate fully with both sets of parents.

Sometimes a non-custodial parent does not take the management of asthma seriously. That parent may not recognize significant triggers and may neglect to give medication on schedule. In other families the custodial parent tries to use asthma as a tool to deprive an ex-spouse of visiting privileges. We try to see that both parents know enough about asthma to provide proper care for their child.

Many of our patients with asthma live in single-parent families. Having a child with chronic asthma is a heavy burden to carry alone. Most single mothers and single fathers in our practice do an excellent job in caring for their children with asthma. They frequently benefit from the support of other parents in similar situations. They cooperate with other single parents in finding solutions to practical problems and making babysitting arrangements. Single parents often bring a friend for support when they attend the Parents' Asthma Group.

For asthma care to proceed smoothly, everyone in the household should be directly and positively involved (see Ryan's story, p. 12). In those families where both the parents know the basics of asthma and the medications used to treat it, there is much less likelihood of overreaction or underreaction to an asthma episode. Asthma is less likely to be used by either a parent or a child in a manipulative way, although we find this to be rare in any case. If all family members have the same understanding and expectations, the demands of asthma care are unlikely to pull them apart.

Six Families

Every family is different and adjusts to asthma in its own way at its own pace. A supportive and accessible physician can speed this process.

Joseph

■

GAIL PLATZ

My son Joseph is five years old and has had occasional asthma episodes since he was one and a half. In August he had a mild episode, and as usual it woke us up at 3:00 A.M. My first response was, maybe it's just croup again, so we steamed up the bathroom for fifteen minutes and tried to read through the fog. Unfortunately that didn't stop the cough or slow his breathing rate down to normal, but he did manage to get back to sleep for a while. I have in my medicine chest an array of medicines but I wasn't sure which one to use or how much. Since it was still the middle of the night I didn't want to wake the doctor, whom I had just met the week before. At last Joey went back to sleep. The following day we took him in to see the doctor, got his medicine straightened out and his asthma under control.

In October we attended the Parents' Asthma Group. Finally, we were learning what was going on and how to deal with it effectively. One of the worst things about the asthma had always been not understanding it. We also learned about the various medications—which are used, how to use them, and perhaps most important, what their effects are. Joey, we discovered, hadn't been taking an effective dose of theophylline and his symptoms would hang on and on. We got a "practice" inhaler and he has now mastered the technique for getting metaproterenol directly into his lungs. We also have a peak flow meter which he can now use correctly although it took him a while to learn.

Perhaps the most valuable part of the parents' asthma group was getting to finally ask all those questions which arise (but you don't feel there is time for) in an office visit, or get forgotten until the next episode. I learned a lot from other people's experiences and how they handled their situations. Another important element was involving both parents in the treatment. This helped me to share the responsibility that I had felt was primarily mine.

In November, Joey had a moderate asthma flare and my husband was the first to notice it. This time everything was easier to deal with since we had a better understanding of what was going on with our son. We were able to bring the flare under control fairly quickly, and with much less anxiety. Joey was soon off to bed and slept peacefully all night.

Michael

■

SHERRY POLITO

My son, Michael, was two years old when he had his first asthma episode. During that time he had a bad cold. I heard some wheezing while he was breathing, and made an appointment to see the doctor. The wheezing got progressively worse and he was having more difficulty breathing. I tried to keep him, and myself, calm. Finally, after receiving three shots of epinephrine, Michael's wheezing subsided. I thought to myself, I don't want Michael to go through this nightmare again. The doctor told me that he definitely had an asthma episode. I shuddered, thinking about what that poor little boy was in for, and wondering how my husband and I could cope with this.

My husband and I are both registered nurses. I worked in a hospital setting for many years and had taken care of many patients with asthma. With all this experience, I was still scared when I heard that Michael had asthma.

Asthma runs on both sides of our family. My husband's sister was very sick with it. My husband remembered how his parents would take her from one doctor to another trying to give her some relief. To this day, his sister is still under treatment. I saw what my parents went through with my brother. He was always so pale and thin and was constantly catching colds. He missed a lot of school due to his asthma. At times he was quite unmanageable. My mother gave in to a lot of his whims, fearing that it would bring on an asthma episode if she were firm.

With all this in mind I didn't want to accept the fact that Michael had asthma. I felt guilty for not bringing him to the doctor's sooner and for thinking the way I did. I felt very nervous wondering how I was going to handle his next attack.

My pediatrician recommended that my husband and I attend an asthma workshop that he was giving. Even when I started the classes I still didn't believe that Michael had asthma. The asthma workshop was quite helpful to us. We were able to share our feelings and listened to others with similar problems and some with more severe problems. The discussion group helped us understand more about asthma and helped us learn when to give Michael the medication he needed.

I didn't want to start medication so late that it wouldn't be effective and I didn't want to give it every time he had a stuffy nose. I was afraid he would have too much theophylline in his system. After the workshop was over, I had a clearer perspective as to how I was going to handle Michael. I was able to cope with his episodes of asthma better. My husband and I both decided that to prevent an flare from getting worse we should treat earlier.

From Michael's asthma records, it seems that Michael goes into his asthma episodes after he catches a cold. Allergies do not affect him so far. We try to prevent his asthma from getting worse by giving him his medication when he starts showing cold symptoms. This has worked for us. We try not to treat Michael any differently than his brother. When Michael is on the medication we let his nursery school teachers know, for he tends to be very high-strung and very active. He is treated just like all the other children and we have had no problems with Michael in nursery school.

We are pleased at the present time with how we are handling Michael's illness. He seems to be doing better now that he is four years old and his trips to the doctor are less frequent.

Christy

■

CECILIA COBBS

Christy is almost four years old. She was born two months prematurely, weighing two pounds, eleven ounces, at birth.

She came home from the hospital two months later. She wasn't breathing normally when she came home. Her lungs were underdeveloped at birth and it was felt that time would strengthen her lungs and the breathing would straighten itself out.

Christy seemed to catch colds easily and with them came difficulty in breathing, more so at night. It was very scary for both of us. The harder it was for her to breathe, the more upset Christy would get and the breathing would become even more difficult. We spent many nights in a rocking chair.

She was about six months old when asthma was first mentioned. I had mixed feelings about asthma. I was relieved to know what the problem was, but also very worried as I knew nothing about it; nor did I know anyone else who had it.

Christy experienced very undesirable side effects from the first couple of drugs she was given. This was very frightening and frustrating. After trying several different drugs we found one that Christy could tolerate.

It seemed that every time she got a cold, the asthma would surface. When Christy was about two years old, she had a prolonged bout with a cold and asthma which required admission to the hospital. I was very scared, I think even more than Christy. She didn't want to stay in the hospital, but we stayed together, which was good for both of us.

Around this time I went to the asthma classes at the doctor's office. This helped me a great deal and ultimately helped Christy. I felt much more relaxed and understood much more about it. It comforted me to listen to other people who understand and deal with the same feelings that I do.

Since attending the sessions, I've found that I don't think about Christy having asthma until it surfaces. Before, I think it was always on my mind and I was constantly waiting for it to happen. The asthma has subsided in the past year. Christy has had fewer colds and hasn't been bothered nearly as much with asthma. And at this point I am very optimistic.

Danny

■

DIANA KOCOT

Danny was just over four when his first episode of asthma occurred. I say episode rather than attack because it was so mild. He had had a cold for what seemed like forever. His baby sitter described his cough as "whistly" the day before we brought him to the doctor. After the doctor listened to Danny's chest and back he asked if I had considered that he might be wheezing. Well, the thought did enter my mind, but I dismissed it quickly. He didn't seem sick enough to have asthma.

The nurse came in and asked Danny to blow into the huffer (peak flow meter). After that he received a treatment with the compressor-driven nebulizer and actually enjoyed it. He held the mouthpiece steady and cooperated really well for the ten-minute treatment. He wanted to know what the medicine was, how it worked and why he needed it. He was fascinated when the nurse showed him diagrams of the windpipes and how they change during an asthma episode. Before we left the doctor showed him how to use an inhaler with the InspirEase holding chamber.

Danny loves to explain his asthma to anyone who wants to know about it. There is no problem in getting him to use his inhaler at home. He acts as though the holding chamber were a toy.

He amazes me with his understanding of asthma. One day when his father lit a cigarette Danny commented, "I'm not going to smoke when I grow up, know why?" When we asked he said, "Because it will bother my asthma and make it worse." We are all very thankful that Danny deals so well with his occasional asthma episodes. Since his comment about cigarettes his father has quit smoking!

Mark

∎

PAT ESPOSITO

Monday night was one of those nights parents dread. Six-year-old Damien awoke at midnight, came into our room and threw up all over me and our bed. By the time we got him cleaned up and back in his own bed two-year-old Mark was wide awake and restless. He didn't fall asleep for another two hours. Mark awoke in the morning with bags under his eyes and "the look." This should have rung an alarm in my head, but I guess I was tired and just not tuned in.

Tuesday, Mark looked a little wiped-out but played happily all day. He went to bed at 7:30 P.M. and fell asleep immediately. At 9:30 P.M. he started coughing a lot. My husband, Bob, and I did a lot of "should we" or "shouldn't we" over whether to start medication. I had treated him for asthma three times the previous winter.

In the midst of this discussion Mark's coughing stopped and he was sleeping peacefully. At close to 1:00 A.M. I was awakened by Mark's coughing and rushed to his room. He had a full expiratory wheeze and was anxious. Since we had missed starting the medicine on time I gave him one-half of a teaspoon of metaproterenol in addition to his long-acting theophylline. The doctor had told me to use it for a severe attack. I had never used it before.

Mark and I then sat in a rocking chair by an open window. I told him that the medicine would help him soon and chatted calmly about other things. Our clock chimed half an hour after I gave him the medicines. By that time Mark's breathing had improved. He was breathing freely and easily and the wheeze gradually disappeared. Although he was still coughing, he became very calm and cheerful and said he felt better.

Mark wasn't able to sleep until after 3:00 A.M. and he awoke coughing again at 6:40 A.M. He took another dose of metaproterenol at 7:00 A.M. and I will give him his second dose of long-acting theophylline at noon. He's having occasional coughing spells but is playing happily and seems comfortable.

This is the first time I have felt confident in diagnosing Mark's problem as asthma without taking him to the doctor. I am sorry I didn't trust my instincts earlier because I could have started the medication much sooner. At the same time I feel elated and grateful that adding the metaproterenol worked so well. I will not be afraid to use it in the future. I also feel pretty confident that the theophylline will begin to help Mark's cough within a few hours as it has in past episodes.

It has taken me a long time to come to terms with the diagnosis of asthma. I kept hoping the problem would disappear. I think I finally accept the fact that Mark has asthma and will on occasion have episodes. Next time I'll start his medicine more promptly.

Mike

■

KATHY BOWLER

The main effect of Mike's asthma on our family is time. When Michael was young and frequently ill, he required a lot of time and attention quite often. I felt I could not go back to work since he was sick during so much (it seemed almost fifty percent) of the fall and winter. When sick, he needed a good deal of attention to keep him calm (some medicines made him awfully shaky), to force fluids, tempt his appetite, keep track of progress and medicines, scratch and rub his back (gets quite itchy), keep him relatively happy (not being able to play with friends is sad), and in general to soothe, comfort, nurse, and get him well.

All this attention and special food and drink for Mike drove his sister into fits of jealousy. The sicker he was, the more attention he required; and the more concern I showed, the more attention she demanded, or tried to demand. For example, we left the children with my mother for a few days. Mike got sick, something my mother was quite competent to handle. She comforted and treated him, and in general was "nurse" for the day. She finally had him settled and quiet in our bed watching television. She got to the dishes, suds up to the elbows, and Cassandra appeared with "let's bake." Mother naturally replied, "Not now, dear." After some wheedling, healthy sister goes and cons the sick one out of bed. Grandmother turned around to see Michael snaking on his stomach, head on pillow, wheezing away, going to play with sister-dear. When I spoke to my mother, she said she could handle Michael; but Cassie, the one she always thought sweet and close to perfect, was driving her mad.

Michael also has numerous food allergies, which require his having different (sister considers them special, better) meals occasionally. Maybe they could be considered special because, if you're making a substitute meal for someone, it's silly to make something they don't like. Well, if you cook special for one, why won't you cook special for two? Why does Cassie have to eat things she doesn't particularly like when Michael doesn't? No amount of talk will convince her that he can't eat it, it will make him sick, but it's good for her. So, you cook special for her, too, sometimes.

Another difference I noted with Michael is that he wasn't invited for dinner or overnight as often as a well child. This seemed to straighten out as he got older. Other mothers were nervous; they did not know what to feed him or what to do if he got sick.

I tried to make it clear that he's just a little boy who is sometimes sick. Not a sickly child. He wanted to do, and could do, the same things as other little boys. He was just as strong and healthy, when not wheezing, as anyone else. Kids with asthma have a bad image.

With specialists, allergy shots, preventatives, emergency visits, check-ups, and medicines for attacks, asthma is not cheap. This also has some effect on the family. Some priorities have to be down-shifted to slip these expenses up on the list.

So, time, keeping child and siblings happy and healthy, and cost are probably, in that order, the main effects on our family of having asthma.

On the positive side, as he's gotten older a good preventive treatment program has been established. I've become aware of the do's and don'ts, and he has also. He's aware of the early signals and is able to initiate early treatment. He is less often ill, requires less time and less special treatment. This eases some of the jealousy from Cassandra. He's happier because he's not missing out on things. His asthma is not important to his peers. It doesn't affect his performance in school or sports. He is accepted for himself.

Holding Chambers Help

Sometimes a parent who knows when to start giving medication and who knows exactly how much to give will be stymied by the most essential step—getting the medication into the patient. There are special pieces of equipment that can help a child to inhale medicine when it is needed most. Two holding chambers, the accordion-style InspirEase, and the bubble-shaped INHAL-AID are described here. (See chapter four for illustrations and instructions).

The InspirEase Works

■

JETTA PELAK

Autumn is Missy's most difficult asthma season. But this year she has not been in to the doctor's office once nor has she missed school. She often starts wheezing and coughing when she plays outdoors in the leaves, but we know that she will get instant relief by using her inhaler with the InspirEase.

I find the InspirEase much more effective than the paper tube. If Missy inhales too rapidly, the "accordion" makes a humming sound and that tells Missy to "slow down." Before we bought the InspirEase, I was never sure that her technique was satisfactory. Another advantage is that she hated using the paper tube but she does not object to using the InspirEase. It's almost a game with her. She thinks it's fun to inflate and deflate the accordion.   ·

Now I can see she is getting the full benefit of her medicine. She stops wheezing and coughing immediately and she's ready to go to school or out to play again after using it. It really has helped us to maintain a normal life and schedule—hassle free.

Michelle and the Bubble

∎

LYNN ARSENEAU

My three-year-old daughter, Michelle, has had asthma since age one. She uses medications continuously, makes many trips to the pediatrician and emergency room, and was hospitalized twice this year. Last fall I heard that we could control her episodes by giving her medication through a metered-dose inhaler. This would replace an office visit for an injection of epinephrine and might prevent admission to the hospital. It would bring her breathing under control and make her episodes less traumatic for everyone.

We bought an inhaler and practiced the routine described on the package insert so we would know how to use it when an episode came. The first time she needed the inhaler, we were visiting my father's farm. The whole family had been looking forward to this weekend of fun and relaxation. Michelle was playing outside when she began having difficulty breathing. She was wheezing and really pulling hard for air. For once I wasn't concerned; I knew the inhaler would save the weekend.

You can probably guess what took place next. My three-year-old started wheezing and was having trouble just trying to take a breath when along comes Mommy with these instructions. "O.K., honey, just stand up, open your mouth wide. I'll hold this thing in front of your mouth, blow out, now I'll spray, you inhale . . . in a steady stream, hold your breath now, 1-2-3-4-5-6-7-8-9-10. Okay, one more time. . . ."

Forget it! The spray went everywhere but down her throat. Some has hit her tongue so she now knows how horrible it tastes. She refuses to try it a second time. Now our child who couldn't breathe is crying, upset and exhausted. Her mother is also crying, upset and exhausted! We head for home, call the doctor, take Michelle in for a long doctor's visit and injections. The weekend is ruined.

If I had known about the Bubble, this scene could have been avoided. The Bubble (INHAL-AID, see p. 114) is a plastic chamber that holds the inhaler spray and allows Michelle to breathe as often as necessary to inhale the spray. She doesn't need exact timing to get the medication into her bronchioles. Because the medication is dispersed into a chamber full of air, it is diluted and there is no bad taste. That really helps!

Even if she can only manage small breaths, the first few will allow enough medication to reach the bronchioles to open those tubes so that the next breaths are deeper. I have noticed this by watching the incentive indicator attached to the mouthpiece. The incentive indicator is a hollow tube with a small plastic "float" inside. The float rises up with each inhalation; the deeper the inhalation, the higher the float rises.

Michelle finds the Bubble very easy to use. A treatment takes only four minutes. The incentive indicator tells me she is getting the medicine into her lungs. I feel more in control. My family is convinced that the Bubble has saved us a lot of difficulty. We don't leave home without it.

Leading a Normal Life

The goal of parents and physicians who are working together to control a child's asthma is not just to keep the child well and out of the hospital, but also to make it possible for a child with asthma to lead a normal life. "Normal" can mean anything from sleeping through the night without coughing to winning a sports trophy. It can mean going to school and keeping up with school work or building up sports skills.

Some of our patients tell what "leading a normal life" means to them.

The Trophy

■

ADRIANNE HALL

I first learned that I had asthma when I was on the swim team in fifth grade. I was always having to slow down in practice and breathe every stroke. My friends were able to swim the length of the pool in just one breath, leaving me far behind. At the time I believed that I was merely out of shape, but our pediatrician suspected otherwise. He heard some wheezes in my chest and said I had mild asthma. My sister and father both have asthma so I was not freaked out. He prescribed theophylline which caused a headache and vomiting. The next time I had trouble with a tight chest he prescribed an adrenergic inhaler. I mastered the inhaler technique, and began seeing results. I thought that was the end of my asthma, but it was not to be the case.

I lost interest in swimming after sixth grade and joined the track team the next year. I had never been much of a sprinter and was in relatively good shape so I figured that my best bet was to run a long distance event. I would practice long and hard, but when it came to running in meets, my time seemed to be stuck at three minutes or above in the 880-yard run and I was never able to place.

It was still the middle of track season when my doctor came by our house to visit with my mother. He asked me how things were going and I mentioned that I was running the half-mile. Then he asked whether I used the inhaler before practice. I told him that I didn't need to, my breathing was fine. He quizzed me some more, "How do you feel at the end of the half mile?" "Just like everybody else," I replied, "they are breathing hard and I am too." "Well," he said, "you might try using your inhaler before practice the next couple of days." I didn't answer him, but the next day I did use it and really felt the difference. Over the next week I cut twenty seconds off of my time. As a result, I was picked to run in the individuals competition in our region of the state. Most importantly, though, I was awarded a huge trophy by the team when they named me the Most Improved Player.

The Tennis Player

■

DAVID PLAUT

Nine years ago when I was nine, I was told that I had asthma. For the first few years I used only an adrenergic inhaler a few times a week and took theophylline tablets two weeks out of the year. Three years ago my asthma problem started getting progressively worse. I now take 800 mg of theophylline a day as well as eight puffs each of albuterol and cromolyn daily. However, I do not consider asthma to be a problem, because it has never prevented me from doing anything I wanted to do.

I have played varsity tennis for three years. I have also played league soccer, basketball, and baseball for a total of fifteen sports seasons. Not once have I missed a game in any sport because of asthma. This is because my asthma is well-controlled. If I did not have an effective treatment plan, I would not have been able to play five hours of tennis daily during the past summer.

Besides taking medications on a regular basis, I use an albuterol inhaler before participating in any sport—even before gym class. Rather than wait for the almost inevitable asthma symptoms to arise in the middle of a game and attempt to subdue them then, my goal is to prevent the symptoms altogether. During the tennis season, using my inhaler has become a regular part of my pre-match routine. I consider it just as basic as stretching or warming-up.

Since I wheeze or get a tight chest when I neglect to pre-treat before exercise, I had to work out a plan that would make it impossible for me to be without my albuterol inhaler. There is always one in my sports bag, in my gym locker, in my house, and in the car. There is no reason to be caught off guard by an asthma flare. Moreover, there is no reason for asthma to prevent anyone from participating in any activity.

You Don't Have to Miss School

■

JETTA PELAK

Last year Melissa, my seven-year-old daughter, had her first asthma attack. She had been rolling in the grass at a soccer field when she broke out in a red, blotchy rash. The next day she complained of sore throat and not feeling well. By early afternoon she was in a deep sleep. She was breathing fifty times a minute and her chest pinched in with every breath.

It was a Sunday and my pediatrician was off-duty. The office of the pediatrician on call was forty-five minutes away so I decided to go to an emergency clinic five minutes from my home. That proved to be a terrible experience. The doctor gave Missy an injection of epinephrine and an inhalation treatment. When we left the clinic she still had retractions. The doctor said there wasn't anything more he could do. It would go away. I certainly didn't know what to do and felt really helpless.

After an hour at home Missy had still not improved. I was shaking as I dialed the pediatrician on call for my doctor. He told me to come to his office immediately. He gave her two more injections and some liquid theophylline to be given every six hours. It took eight days until Missy felt well enough to return to school.

About five weeks later Melissa had another attack, after a field trip in the woods with her Brownie Troop. We met her pediatrician in his office at 11:00 P.M. He gave her two injections of epinephrine and said Missy definitely had asthma. He prescribed liquid theophylline to be taken for seven days. After that, she was to take long-acting theophylline every eight hours and cromolyn three times a day. Missy improved slowly and returned to school after six days.

Six weeks ago we moved to Western Massachusetts and into a very old and damp house. Since the move, Missy has had a cough at night and wakes up with terrible nasal congestion. She recently saw a doctor for her school physical. He said she was in good health. I mentioned her asthma symptoms and he suggested that I consider discontinuing the theophylline. He also recommended that I use a metaproterenol inhaler along with the cromolyn and read a book called *Children With Asthma*.

I couldn't consider any of these changes since it seemed to me that Melissa needed the theophylline more than ever. I did buy the book that week and began to read it, and at the same time made an appointment with an asthma specialist. Four weeks before the scheduled appointment Melissa woke up on a Sunday with a very bad cough. She complained of chest pain, shortness of breath, and a sore throat. I took her to the doctor who prescribed an albuterol inhaler. Somehow I had the same helpless feeling as I left that office. It just didn't seem like enough.

That night was horrible. She went into that deep sleep again as she had with her first attack. She was breathing thirty-six times per minute and her stomach pushed out with each breath. It was an effort for her to breathe in and out. I sat on her bed with a flashlight all night and counted her respirations every hour, praying that we could make it until morning.

Several times I got up to wake my husband to take us to the emergency room at the hospital. But I was afraid to go there, too. The albuterol inhaler proved useless to Melissa. Her chest hurt too much to take a deep breath. When she needed it the most (during the middle of the night) I couldn't wake her enough to sit up, let alone coordinate her breathing with the inhaler puff.

Finally morning came. I called the asthma specialist's office and arranged to see him. I was sure he would give her an injection to make her breathe easier. Melissa was scared when we were taken into the treatment room. The doctor's assistant told her that this doctor did not like to give children needles.

The doctor explained the four signs of asthma trouble to me while he was examining Melissa. He told me to watch for a change in her wheezing, retractions, prolonged expiration, and respiratory rate as she received the treatment. Then he went out to see another patient while the nurse measured metaproterenol and saline into a plastic nebulizer unit. She turned on the air compressor and a mist came out of the mouthpiece. She asked Melissa to hold the mouthpiece between her teeth and to breathe in and out. I saw a big improvement in Missy's breathing about two minutes after she started breathing in the mist.

The entire treatment lasted about eight minutes. Half an hour later, the nurse watched as I gave Missy the next treatment. Her peak flow rate had been 60 when we arrived. After two treatments it was 200. I borrowed the compressor-driven nebulizer to use at home every four hours. The doctor also prescribed prednisone for three days and said to continue the theophylline as before and to give metaproterenol and cromolyn by nebulizer.

That evening Melissa had two more treatments at home while watching television. Her breathing was peaceful that night. The doctor called to check on her at 8:00 P.M. and I felt more reassured than I ever have. I knew I could fall asleep and not worry. The next morning she continued taking four medications: metaproterenol and cromolyn by nebulizer, long-acting theophylline, and prednisone. She did some arts and crafts, made pudding for herself and her brother, and balleted around the house. I received another call at 4:00 P.M. from the doctor's office to check on her progress. That follow-up meant a lot to me.

The next morning she took her medicine. Then we had breakfast and went out to walk the dog. Missy and her dog ran far ahead of me up the hill. I was out of breath, but Missy was not. I brought Missy to school with her nebulizer and arranged for a health aide to give her a treatment at noon. When I picked her up at the end of the day, she was feeling fine.

This time was different. I learned a lot and I know I'm going to learn much more. But the big difference is that it only took twenty-four hours for Melissa to recover. Now I have a written plan and know what to do. When the next episode comes, I will be ready for it.

Twenty Years of Coughing Asthma

■

BETH GRADONE

Every time I got a cold, I coughed. Endlessly. But I never, ever wheezed. I thought every kid coughed for months after they had colds. Twenty years ago, when I was a nine year old living in the suburbs of Boston, no one knew that asthma could cause a chronic cough. Every winter of my childhood found the family vaporizer by my bed and all kinds of concoctions for suppressing coughs in the family medicine cabinet.

None of it ever worked. I'm told I coughed in my sleep, when I fell asleep at all. From November to April, I frequently slept sitting up all night to avoid the tight-chested cough. I remember taking codeine cough syrup in college. The combination of codeine and lack of sleep at night made it impossible for me to stay awake during the day. My roommate took notes for me when I slept through lectures.

In November 1983 my usual cold and cough started, then the cold subsided and the cough stayed on. This time the cough worsened until one Saturday night my chest was so tight I didn't know if I'd be able to keep breathing until the morning. The next day, I went to see the doctor. Even at this stage I hadn't figured out what I was dealing with. I only knew every breath hurt, and trying just to speak made me cough uncontrollably.

Fortunately, even though the doctor didn't hear a wheeze, she suggested a trial of metaproterenol mist. Within minutes I started to feel better and by the end of the treatment I felt normal. She prescribed a metaproterenol inhaler for me to use at home. Getting my timing right with the inhaler was tough; I still use a paper tube as a holding chamber for the mist. I always carry the inhaler with me. It is the only asthma medicine I need.

My diagnosis is mild asthma. I've figured out that my main trigger is an upper respiratory infection with post-nasal drip. I get one every fall. When I cough to clear my throat, I sometimes trigger asthma symptoms.

I discovered that exercise and cold air also trigger episodes. One day this past winter I was feeling fine and didn't (for once) have a respiratory infection when I had to run hard to get to a concert on time. I made it but my chest was tight and I was dying to use my inhaler through the whole concert. Right afterward two puffs from the inhaler brought me immediate relief.

Thinking back, I remember having a hard time keeping up with my karate class in the winter. We met in a large but cold room. I coughed and was short of breath all the time. I had thought I was "out of shape." Since I started taking proper medication for asthma, coughing is not a problem and I now can get a good night's sleep.

Some Principles for Managing Asthma

■

JOE DUFFY

I have the distinct advantage of writing this narrative about a year after reading my wife's story of our son, Matthew, in chapter one. Matthew is eight years old now and is a happy, healthy, outgoing, well-adjusted, athletic child with budding interests in rock 'n roll, fast cars, baseball, and junk food. Until maybe a year ago, however, if someone asked, "How's Matt?" the status of his asthma would probably have emerged early in the answer and received considerable emphasis. In fact, the qualities I just described—the qualities that represent what Matt really is—sometimes were never mentioned or were given only token attention. Today, asthma is often not part of the answer at all. Today, the short answer to that question is usually "Good."

A number of things have reduced the importance of asthma in our lives. First, Jeamie and I have become good observers of behaviors which signal that Matt's asthma is active to an extent which requires close watching, an increase or change in medication, or a call or visit to his doctor. When it becomes active, one must treat it aggressively enough to restore breathing function to "normal" or keep to it in check until the triggering event (cold, weather, allergen, etc.) is no longer present. Arriving at this understanding was of major importance in our adjustment to, and treatment of, Matt's asthma. When Matt was between one and three years old, I very often reacted to the beginning of an asthma episode with a kind of denial. I attributed his wheezing or coughing to a cold or some other cause and assumed that the symptoms would simply not last or worsen. This attitude often delayed treatment and sometimes resulted in the episode becoming worse than it needed to be. Today, we're good at recognizing when symptoms or behavior are asthma related and we take action as soon as possible.

Secondly, Jeamie and I have learned as much about asthma as is necessary for us to play an active role in its management. We do not accept the notion that the physician is the only person capable of accurately observing and managing asthma in our child. We believe that the parents and the patient are almost always in a better position to observe the onset and progression of symptoms and the effect of treatment, both long before and long after the physician has examined the child. We have been extremely fortunate to have pediatricians whose philosophy of asthma care involves the parents' becoming active partners in treatment.

Under this philosophy of management, a lot of work is required. This "work," for us, has included reading and learning facts about the nature of asthma; learning what its symptoms are; learning how to reliably recognize those symptoms and their meaning; learning the purpose of medications and their intended results and negative side effects; learning the purpose and meaning of measuring blood levels for theophylline; learning to estimate in to out ratios and breathing rates; learning how to report relevant facts to the physician or nurse; and, perhaps most importantly, learning how to ask questions, without embarrassment, which will contribute to future management of asthma problems. All of this learning has taken years but the results have been rewarding. For us, knowledge is not only power but it also reduces our anxiety and fear about a problem that need not be the unknowable monster many people perceive it to be.

The last factor which has been important in managing Matt's asthma deals with our relationship with him. We have tried our best to mark our relationship with calmness, confidence, honesty, education, and an absence of rewards for being sick. Calmness and confidence are strongly tied to one another. We are able to be calm during asthma episodes (even those necessitating hospitalization) because we recognize his symptoms and their meaning and because we understand the reasons for the treatment that he receives. We're able to tell Matt why we're asking certain questions ("Do you feel wheezy?"), or observing his breathing rate, or listening for wheezing. We can tell him why we're doing the things that we find necessary to manage the problem (increase medication or fluid intake, visit the doctor, or go to the hospital). At such times, I know the ability to be calm and confident makes Jeamie and me feel good about ourselves. I'm sure that our calmness and confidence reduces any "fear of the unknown" that Matt might have and minimizes the role that anxiety might play in increasing the severity of the episode. We've really begun to see the payoff of this approach in the last two years—Matt is now at least as calm as we are during an episode.

We've also learned that honesty and education about the problem really pays off in terms of Matt's realism and calmness about his asthma. For example, if we need to see a doctor during an episode, we tell him he may have to have a shot and that it will hurt a bit—in fact, shots are amazingly routine now because he gets two allergy shots every Friday. When hospitalization has been necessary we've told him that we are going before we got there, why, and what would be done when we arrived. The last time he was hospitalized, he told *us* what probably would be done, and he was right! To the best of our ability, we also answer any questions he asks, such as: Why do I have asthma? Will I always get allergy shots? Will I always have asthma? What does this pill do? When we can't answer a question, he is encouraged to ask his doctor or nurse when he sees them next.

We place a minimum of restrictions on his physical activities, even when he is wheezy. The exceptions to this involve avoidance of known major allergens for Matt. For example, he can't go to a barn down the road because he's very allergic to the horses there. We've discovered that Matt has always been a good judge of what he should and shouldn't do physically. If he's quite wheezy and plays soccer, he'll often quit in just a short time. We always try to encourage physical and athletic activity, but balance it by acknowledging his good common sense to quit when it's appropriate. We have tried to minimize the attention we pay to his asthma during our daily routines: medicine gets put on the table to be taken, not talked about; allergy shots are an in-and-out-of-the-doctor's-office-as-soon-as-possible event. Asthma is a topic of conversation only if Matt raises the issue.

I think all of these things have helped us and Matt to think of him not as "an asthmatic" but as a youngster who just happens to have asthma, just like other people have warts, colds, arthritis, and hemorrhoids. It's part of what he is, and it deserves a degree of attention. But it's only a small part and, hopefully, not very important to how people view him or his ultimate achievements.

Our present attitudes and beliefs about Matt's asthma are colored by the relatively long period of time in which we have not had to deal with major episodes. After nearly eight years of experience we have learned to deal with Matt's asthma effectively.

Babysitters and Others

As you know, most neighbors, babysitters, and relatives have little knowledge of asthma. What do they need to know about asthma in order to interact properly with your child? The amount of information you give will depend on the severity and frequency of flares, the amount of time your child spends in their care, and the availability of people who can help in case of a problem.

A babysitter should have some general knowledge about asthma as outlined in "What is Asthma?" (see chapter two). The sitter should also have specific information about medications: time and method of administration, desired effects, and side effects. Instructions about whom to call in case of an asthma flare are essential. Adequate instruction for a babysitter or an overnight visit can be supplied by filling in the form below.

Neighbors and children who are in contact with but not responsible for your child should understand that asthma does not usually interfere with normal activity. Interested adults should have the opportunity to read, "What is Asthma?" and discuss your child's status with you.

Instructions for the Babysitter

_____ has asthma.
He/she takes the following medicines on a regular basis:
adrenergic inhaler, as

_____, a double whiff every four hours
with an attack.
theophylline, as _____ mg
at _____ and _____.

If _____ has a peak flow score
under _____ or has difficulty breathing and:
___ makes a noise breathing out
___ sucks in the chest skin
___ takes longer to breathe out than breathe in
___ breathes faster than usual
___ complains of a tight chest
___ _____

please call me for instructions at _____. If you cannot reach me,
call Dr. _____ at _____.
Please see attached sheets for more information on asthma, medications, and when to give them.

6
School and Travel

School

Our schools are trying to do a good job of educating our children. Obviously, absences interfere with a student's learning. Sporadic absences are particularly disruptive. We try to keep children in school as much as possible. This means that they return to school during an asthma flare and do not miss class for minor episodes.

Asthma flares do occur in school. The school staff needs explicit instructions if they are to respond appropriately. In this chapter you will read of a teenager who kept her asthma a secret and had problems with a flare. After good communication between her mother and the principal, she was able to handle future episodes effectively. Sample instructions for a school nurse are presented.

Teachers should know about asthma in order to react properly to the students' complaints. An "Information Form for Teacher" outlines the situation. Often a child with asthma can give a report to inform his or her class about this common problem. In the process, the student will learn more about asthma and may become better able to control it.

A student often has to take medication during the school day to keep an asthma flare under control. In addition, his or her activity may have to be temporarily reduced.

What is a proper medication policy for a school? We believe that all junior and senior high school students should be able to carry and regulate their own medication. It is too cumbersome and embarrassing for them to check in with the school nurse for each dose of medicine. However, a record of all drugs a student is taking should be on file in the health office.

In general, elementary school students should go to the nurse's room for medication. This will cut down on abuse of the inhaler, and also insure that the medication is taken at the proper time. Those students who are responsible enough to take their medicine as directed should be allowed to do so. This may be negotiated between parent, school nurse, and doctor.

We try to arrange medication schedules so that a minimum of medication is taken during school hours. The adrenergic inhaler is used every four hours during an episode. If it is used before school, it should not be used more than twice during the school day. It should be available to prevent exercise-induced asthma. Theophylline usually can be taken every twelve hours and usually is not taken during school hours. Administration of cromolyn and prednisone can usually be spaced to avoid the school day.

Teachers need guidance from parents to decide when a student should be kept inside, excused from gym, sent to the nurse's room, and under what circumstances a parent should be notified of an asthma problem.

Each of these situations can be anticipated. If the school staff receive explicit instructions they perform very well. For an example of one school's response to a problem, see the account of Monica's episode and the subsequent correspondence between her mother and the principal.

The school health staff in the Amherst school system raised the following questions during an in-service program:

How do you relieve anxiety in a child who is having an attack?

The school nurse must have a written plan of action supplied by the parent for taking care of an asthma episode. It should include quiet talk, administration of warm liquids, administration of medications as prescribed and contact with the parent if improvement is not prompt.

How do you deal with gym teachers who either don't believe that a child is having trouble, or who restrict the child's activities when it doesn't seem necessary?

Gym teachers spend a lot of time dealing with students who prefer rest to exercise. Ideally, the parent and doctor will have defined, in writing, the circumstances in which the student should be excused from gym. Peak flow rate can serve as an objective guide for this decision. Most children with asthma can participate fully in gym except during a flare at which time their activities should be scaled down. Children with exercise-induced asthma should use an adrenergic or cromolyn inhaler before gym to prevent problems.

What do you do with a medication that is not properly labelled?

Medications must be labeled with name, strength, amount to be given, and the time of administration. Inadequately labelled medicine should be returned to the parent for proper labelling.

What are the side effects of the various medications?

The most troublesome side effect for the school staff is the hyperactivity produced by theophylline in some children. This can often be lessened by using a sustained released theophylline preparation or by adding an adrenergic drug or cromolyn to the treatment plan.

What can be done about students who start wheezing in cold weather when traveling to school?

The student can wear a surgeon's mask or a painter's mask. This creates a reservoir of warm air and thus reduces the amount of cold air reaching the bronchioles. Of course, most kids wouldn't be caught dead wearing one of these masks unless it is hidden by a scarf.

Monica's Attack

■

MONICA CYRAN

It was Friday and ever since second period gym, I was having a hard time breathing, but I was too busy and too embarrassed to go and use my inhaler between classes. We only have three minutes to run to our lockers and get our books for next period. By the time fifth period English came, I realized I'd better get my inhaler or die on the spot. That's when I went to my teacher, to ask for a pass to my locker. Of course she said no. I had tried to get out of her classes before. She yelled at me and said I should go sit because I had tried to get out and visit my friends during first period lunch (this is normally true, but this time it was different).

I asked her a second time if I could go to my locker and get my inhaler. She screamed no again. She was especially grouchy because there were so many people around her desk. By that time, if she didn't let me go, I was gonna go without her permission and worry about it later. Then I thought, she already hates me anyway, I'd better try one more time. So I screamed at her, "I have asthma." (It took just about everything I had to say this.) "I have to get my inhaler, I'm having an attack." "Go, go, go ahead!!! I don't care what you do anyway!" So I booked.

While running down three flights of stairs to get to the freshmen lockers in the basement (they make us start at the bottom), I thought I'd never make it there. I was having a hard time breathing. I know that sounds dramatic, but I felt lousy!

I got there and just really wanted that medicine in my lungs so I could feel better. I felt so dizzy. Just then the nurse's aide saw me and brought me to her office. She sat me down and I was so weak I fell down and I passed out. All that was because I do not bother to carry my inhaler—I know I should. Also, I took my medicine carelessly. It's too late now to say what I should have done, but everyone says, you learn valuable lessons from dumb mistakes.

Letter to Monica's Principal

Dear Mr. Murray:

On Friday, October 8, 1982, Monica had an asthma attack during her English class. She attempted three times to ask her teacher if she might leave and get the inhaler she kept in her locker. By the time she did get to her locker, she was weak. It was fortunate she was near the teachers' room when someone noticed she wasn't feeling well. She was assisted into the room, and helped. By this time it was too late for her to make a quick recovery using the inhaler. She had to come home from school.

I would like to know if there is some way that all of her teachers could be notified that Monica has asthma, and from time to time needs to use her inhaler. I have attached a note from her doctor verifying the fact that she uses the inhaler. You will see that it is dated August 30, 1982. Monica did not feel the need to bring it in before this incident.

I realize that it is hard for teachers to comply with students' wishes every time they want to leave the classroom. In fairness to her teachers, I would expect to be notified if a teacher felt Monica was abusing this request.

Any help you can offer will be greatly appreciated. If you feel a conference is necessary, please let me know.

Thank you in advance for your cooperation.

Sincerely,

Celine Cyran

Letter from Principal

PALMER HIGH SCHOOL
24 CONVERSE STREET
PALMER, MASSACHUSETTS 01069

October 13, 1982

Mrs. Celine Cyran
186 Shearer Street
Palmer, Massachusetts

Dear Mrs. Cyran:

This letter is relative to your correspondence of October 11, 1982 concerning Monica's asthmatic condition.

Be assured we will make every one of Monica's teachers aware of her chronic condition. On Friday, October 8th, no one in the school was aware of the situation and as a result of it, the same rules and regulations were applied to Monica as to all other students. It wasn't until she made the teacher aware of her condition that she was allowed to leave the classroom.

As of today each of her teachers will be totally aware of her situation.

Sincerely yours,

Alphonse E. Murray, Jr.
Principal

M/b

COMMENT: Monica is a typical teenager. She did not want the embarrassment of being tagged as having asthma so she didn't give my note to the school nurse. Thus, the school had no knowledge of her problem. The school administration and staff are now informed of her status and will respond appropriately.

INFORMATION FOR SCHOOL NURSE

Please use this form as a sample for a letter informing the school nurse what to expect of your child. I suggest that you fill it out, then copy it over to avoid confusion about the items which do not apply.

_____ has asthma. Ordinarily he/she can be as active as any other child and should not have his/her activities restricted in any way. During a flare, he/she should not go out in the cold or engage in strenuous physical activity.

_____ takes the following medicines in school at the times noted:

____ albuterol/metaproterenol by inhaler at _____ and _____.

____ theophylline as _____ mg at _____.

____ cromolyn at _____.

____ He/She uses the inhaler before sports or if he/she is wheezing during physical activity.

____ He/She should _____ carry his/her inhaler all the time, _____ leave it

in a locker, _____ keep it in the health room.

____ knows when he/she needs his/her inhaler—please let him/her use his/her judgment. He/She is not to use it more than once in a school day unless I have written you a note.

Please let me know if you would like a fuller description of his/her medicines.

I will be glad to give you the handouts which his/her doctor has written and to go over them with you.

In case you have questions, please call me at home at _____

or at work _____.

If you can't reach me, please call _____

at _____who knows what to do. If that fails,

please call his/her doctor, Dr. _____, at _____ for advice.

Sincerely,

_____

INFORMATION FOR TEACHER

Please use this form as a sample for a letter informing the teacher what to expect of your child. I suggest that you fill it out, then copy it over to avoid confusion about the items which do not apply.

_____ has asthma.

Ordinarily, he/she can be as active as any other child and should not have his/her activities restricted in any way.

During a flare, he/she should not go out in the cold or engage in strenuous physical activity.

The medicine which he/she takes occasionally causes headaches and stomach aches and can make him/her jumpy.

Please let me know if you consider his/her behavior inappropriate. He/She should not be allowed to misbehave any more than any other kid in the class.

I have left a list of medicines which he/she takes with the school nurse. I would like to discuss

_____'s asthma with you.

I hope that _____ will be able to give a report on asthma to his/her class. He/She knows a lot about it and we find that his/her friends are interested in hearing how it all works.

Sincerely,

_____

ADMINISTRATION OF MEDICATION IN SCHOOL

The goal of treatment is to allow the child with asthma to lead a normal and fully active life. When parents, physicians, the school nurse and the patient work together, they can almost always achieve this goal. The administration of theophylline, cromolyn and prednisone can usually be scheduled to fall outside school hours. Inhaled adrenergic drugs must be taken at closer time intervals. In addition, they are often taken before gym or participation in a sports program. Some children need to use a compressor-driven nebulizer to treat an asthma episode. Without it, they would miss school (see p. 166). The statement below, by the Committee on School Health of the American Academy of Pediatrics*, gives guidelines which can lead to safe and responsible administration of medication in the school.

Many children with chronic disabilities or illnesses are able to attend school because of the effectiveness of their prescribed medication. Any student who is required to take prescribed medication during regular school hours should do so in compliance with school regulations. These regulations should include the following:

1. A physician should provide written orders with the name of the drug, dose, time interval when the medication is to be taken, and diagnosis or reason the medicine is needed.

2. The parent or guardian should provide a written request that the school district comply with the physician's order.

3. Medication should be brought to school in a container appropriately labeled by the pharmacist or the physician.

4. When the student does not regularly take his or her own medication, or if the parent or physician requests that school personnel administer the medication, provision should be made for the medication to be kept in a locked cabinet. Designated personnel must be available to administer the medication at agreed-upon times, and arrangements should be made for alternate personnel to perform the task in case of absence. The person administering the medication must keep a written record.

5. When the child is usually responsible for taking his/her own medication, he/she may do so in school without supervision by school personnel, provided the physician and parent have provided the

*PEDIATRICS, vol. 74: 433, Copyright © 1984. Used with permission.

required authorizations. The school administration should cooperate with the physician, parent, and child. In such instances, it is understood that the school bears no responsibility for safeguarding the medication or assuring that it is taken, and the parent should provide a written statement relieving the school of such responsibility.

6. Individual school districts should seek the advice of counsel as they assume the responsibility for giving medication during school hours. Liability coverage should be provided for the staff including nurses, teachers, athletic staff, principals, superintendents, and members of the school board.

It would be wise to meet with the school nurse to discuss your child's treatment plan. Many nurses are willing to monitor peak flow rates as well as to give medicine. If the nurse fully understands your child's asthma program, she will be able to provide efficient assistance in the case of an asthma episode. In addition, her observations will help you to insure that your child will rarely miss school because of asthma.

Travel

Parents need a plan to deal with asthma episodes that occur while their child is away from home. Written instructions are even more important in this situation than when you are in familiar surroundings.

Emily: The Thanksgiving Disaster

■

GAIL HALL

When my brother phoned to ask us to join his family for Thanksgiving dinner, I was delighted. I was very ready to take a break from combining work, school, and single parenthood, even if it was only for two days. I think I would have been glad to go anywhere as long as it took me out of Amherst, but I was especially happy for a chance to enjoy my sister-in-law's fantastic cooking and to visit their new baby. Yet I couldn't help feeling some misgiving. On our last visit to New York City my six-year-old daughter, Emily, had an asthma reaction to my brother's cats and we had spent Easter dinnertime in the emergency room.

Emily had been diagnosed as having asthma three years earlier. Most of the trouble occurred as a result of infection; when she got a cold, she got asthma. Trouble with allergies was something fairly new. I'd learned a lot about keeping Emily well in my own home, but I hadn't really become comfortable with travel and the demands it made on me. One of the things I liked the least was imposing the asthma situation on other people's lives. I knew that in preparation for our visit my brother and sister-in-law would do a lot of extra vacuuming and cleaning to try to get rid of the cat hairs. They told me on the phone that they had kept the cats out of the guest room since summer. But even with these preparations, I knew I would still have to pay constant close attention to Emily, and hoped my monitoring wouldn't dominate everyone else's experience of the visit. I knew I would find it difficult to say, "Oh, excuse me, let me just listen to her breathing here," or, "I wonder where she is in the house." I imagined myself walking in the door saying, "Hi! So glad to see you. Could we put this rug somewhere else? Is your humidifier working?"

I planned for trouble as best I could. I let my brother know that I wouldn't make the final decision about coming until the last minute. If Emily developed a cold we would have to cancel our trip since I knew that a cold would send her over the edge if she were with cats. Three days before we were scheduled to leave I put her on the metaproterenol inhaler. I increased her dose gradually, from one day to the next, until she was using it three times a day, two whiffs each time. This gradual approach helps prevent adverse effects. I decided to use the inhaler, even though I knew it was likely that I would be getting up two or three times during the night, because she doesn't sleep well when she's taking the inhaler. That was just part of the deal. I also let my brother know that it was likely to be a very brief trip.

On Thanksgiving Day we took the bus to New York and arrived at my brother's before noon. After lunch and a turn holding my baby niece, I helped Emily with her midday medications. We were able to tell fairly quickly that things might not go as smoothly as we wanted. I didn't have a peak flow meter, but had developed my own system of gauging Emily's ability to breathe. It's important to hold your breath after using the inhaler so that the medication gets absorbed. But if you are heading into trouble with asthma, your breathing gets faster and holding your breath gets harder and harder. Emily took the first whiff from the inhaler and tried to hold her breath while I counted out loud, "One green elephant, two green elephants . . ." We only made it to four. After the second whiff, we got as far as six. The difficulty she had holding her breath let me know that Emily was reacting to the environment.

So I knew we were having some difficulty. I could have tuned into the situation more clearly at that point and decided it was time to leave, but I really didn't want to. I told myself that perhaps I had miscounted, or perhaps the inhaler would see us through anyway, along with the long-acting theophylline that she took twice a day. My brother and sister-in-law had washed the guest room walls, vacuumed the rugs within an inch of their lives, and placed a new humidifier in the center of the room. The rest of the house was also spotless, as always, and the turkey was filling the house with its promise of an irreplaceable family feast. It was definitely not the time to go home.

The rest of the day was the kind of balancing act I had feared it would be. When I took the suitcases upstairs to the guest room, it was indeed moist and clean, right down to the tenacious cat hairs which my all too wary eye detected. I kept an eye on Emily, shooed her away from the cats, and tried to limit her time with the dog she adored. After a while I sent her upstairs to the guest room to watch television. After our Thanksgiving dinner, the second use of the inhaler told me things were a little worse. When asked, Emily said she was fine. As far as Emily is concerned, what is ignored will go away. I began to think of ways to stay out of the house the next day.

The next morning Emily was having so much trouble breathing that even my sister-in-law knew Emily was fibbing when she said she was fine. As we worked on the second round of the

Thanksgiving dishes, we devised a plan for getting everyone out of the house and on the road, in hopes of giving Emily's breathing a chance to get back to normal. The weather was nice enough to go to the Bronx Zoo, so we got people fed and left for the day. We'd be outside, and everyone, including Emily's eleven-year-old sister, Adrianne, could have a good time. I was being a little too optimistic, however. The event could have been entitled "The Salvation Army Goes to the Zoo." Emily was having so much trouble breathing that she had difficulty walking up the hills the zoo provided. My brother carried her while Adrianne limped along behind in the leg brace she was wearing for her troublesome but not serious knee problem, chondromalacia of the patella. I watched the clock, trying to decide whether to leave enough time for a trip to my sister's pediatrician if things didn't improve. But we were having a good time and I figured the worst that could happen if we stayed was an evening trip to the emergency room as we had done last Easter. On that trip she received a shot of Sus-Phrine, a long-acting form of epinephrine got us through the night. So we stayed at the zoo and I was glad to see Adrianne having a good time while we forgot as best we could about asthma for awhile.

At five o'clock everyone was tired. We used the inhaler again, but things weren't getting better. In fact, they were getting worse. The inhaler ceased being useful because Emily could no longer hold her breath long enough to let the medication stay in the bronchial tubes and have its effect. In a last effort to play for time, I suggested we go for ice cream. Of course, any fool who decides to stop and get something to eat in New York gets what she deserves. There were no ice cream parlors anywhere. My brother didn't know ice cream parlors; his kid was only four months old. Emily was getting exhausted and Adrianne was beginning to show signs of wear and tear. She had realized that things had turned and we were now "doing asthma." So every time we got in and out of the car looking for ice cream, she followed Emily into the back seat with "You little jerk, you're faking it." The third time she did, I offered to punch her in the mouth. The situation had deteriorated.

From then on events progressed pretty quickly. We did manage to find a delicatessen. Emily, now without an appetite, managed to eat some jello and Adrianne enjoyed some New York cheesecake. I let my brother know that things were definitely not okay and we left for his house, not really sure what to do. We arrived at home and I sent Emily up to the guest room. I wanted a minute to rest and think and I thought this room was the best place in the house for her to be. But I was wrong. Unbeknownst to me, Emily was allergic to more than just cat hairs. There were other things in the room to which she reacted. Within minutes she was in severe distress. Adrianne came downstairs and told me Emily was really sick. I said I knew she was sick and I was planning to come upstairs in a few minutes. Her real concern for her sister came through as she made it totally clear that we were needed upstairs NOW. She played a crucial role here, since it would have been extremely difficult at this point for Emily to walk down the stairs and ask for help. I wrapped Emily in a blanket while my brother got the car started. We drove to the hospital with Emily lying in the back seat, gasping short breaths, no longer pretending she was okay.

We drove to the hospital in Bronxville where we had been at Easter. The same doctor who was there in April was not there now, of course, and things looked pretty busy in the emergency room. I brought Emily in and after the usual insurance procedures I told the nurse that Emily was having trouble with asthma, that I thought she needed an injection, that we had been there before, that she took theophylline, a 200 mg tablet twice a day, and that she used a metaproterenol inhaler, but it was no longer useful to us because she was unable to hold her breath.

The nurse spoke with the intern or resident and he came over and asked me what I thought the problem was. I repeated what I had said to the nurse and added that I felt that, given Emily's previous experience with asthma, the situation warranted an injection of adrenalin. "I think she needs a shot because the oral medication we've been using is no longer working," I said. "I think you need to calm down," was his response.

I had entered the emergency room aware that I had to play a

low key role because I knew some physicians found it difficult to deal with parents who have a lot of information, and, God help them, an opinion. I understood that it was important to avoid acting as if I were going to be the one to make a decision. Instead, it was my role to simply feed information, and very slowly at that. I understood it was important not to irritate the people who had the drug my kid needed. In retrospect, I see that I should have followed this insight more closely and not suggested the shot. At any rate, I was not prepared for the level of hostility that I met, partly because it was not there on my last visit, and partly because I am never prepared for hostility.

We had to wait another fifteen minutes for the physician who was on-duty. He was moving from bed to bed and it seemed that he had spoken with the nurse and the intern or resident. The fact that it was hard to tell who was who or who had talked with whom illustrates a device that I think people either consciously or subconsciously use in emergency rooms. That is, no one identifies themselves in terms of rank or name. They simply move at you and away from you without letting you know who they are, who is making decisions, what's going on, or what the plan is. He finally came over and listened very briefly to Emily's chest. His diagnosis was, "This isn't an asthma attack." As he walked away with an air of disdain, he remarked over his shoulder, "She's hyperventilating."

I was amazed that he did not notice her retractions or that her inhale to exhale ratio was reversed, two signs of real trouble with breathing. They occur with asthma, but not with hyperventilation. I knew why he said she wasn't having an asthma attack. It was because she wasn't wheezing. But wheezing isn't an essential part of an asthma attack; in fact, you can only wheeze if some air goes through the windpipes. Emily wasn't wheezing because many of her windpipes were completely closed.

I started to say something but he was gone. I was trying to hold out for a rational explanation for what was going on, but it was difficult. Perhaps the emergency room was truly overloaded with emergencies; however, all I had heard were two discussions of how to apply ace bandages and where to go for a throat culture. While the physician was gone, the nurse gave Emily oxygen through a nasal device. He returned, after another fifteen minutes, and took the device off Emily, saying, "We don't need this." He started firing questions at me about her medications and interrupting me every time I tried to answer. Finally he said, "We'll give her an injection. We can x-ray her, too." After more delays and confusion she got the injection and x-rays. To no one's surprise, she did not have pneumonia. As we left, I said to myself that even though it had been a truly unpleasant experience, it was over. We were home free. She would sleep through the night as she had done at Easter and we would leave right away in the morning.

We went back to my brother's house and I put Emily to bed. Soon thereafter, I went to sleep in the room with her. What I thought would be a night of much-needed sleep turned into a nightmare. Emily woke at midnight in real distress and beginning to panic. She was struggling to catch her breath with little success. The inhale to exhale ratio was reversed. She was exhaling with such difficulty that it sounded like somebody was punching her in the stomach every time she tried to exhale. I was becoming upset because I couldn't help her and things weren't making any sense. Also, I was going to have to get my brother out of bed and go back out in the cold.

When we got back to the emergency room, the intern, I could see, was not pleased to see us but somewhat softened in his response. The other physician was gone for the night. The nurses were solicitous as usual and trying to be useful. I came with the fear that the intern would decide that the next step would be to give Emily more injected medication. On several occasions when she had had more than one shot in one day she had developed severe side effects. While most kids get cranky and nervous, Emily gets paranoid. She imagines that she is in danger, that everything around her is rotting. Her legs shake. She has fits of anger. It usually starts with a headache, pain in her chest and vomiting, and lasts for an hour or more. In short, a bad drug trip. I had gotten used to the vomiting—vomiting on the sidewalk is part of living with asthma—but I had never gotten used to that terror.

I went in to the emergency room thinking about how I would have to deal with people who really didn't want to see me again. Last time, I just had to wait it out until they gave her the medicine. This time I was going to have to try to change their minds. I wanted them to admit her to the hospital, and give her medicine intravenously. When she had been hospitalized in October, oxygen and intravenous medication had brought the breathing under control and there had been no side effects. Also, if she were in the hospital she would be away from the cats, which had been the source of the problem. Even though at that time I didn't know how her allergy situation had changed, I knew *something* had changed. I knew I couldn't go back to my brother's house.

I presented my case to the intern: "I don't think she should have another injection. I know from my experience with injections that it might cut the symptoms in half at best, and—I don't know for sure—but she may have severe side effects which, given how uncomfortable she is now, seems like a bad idea." "Well, who's the doctor here?" shouted the resident or intern or whoever he was. I said, "I can tell you from my experience that we're not going to have any success with just injections. I can't go home. I either have to go to a motel room in the middle of the night or she has to spend the night in the hospital." "Well," he said, "we'll have to call in the pediatrician who is on call." I felt bad, I don't know why, about getting somebody else out of bed on a cold night.

The pediatrician came in about half an hour later and said, "Have you had this child desensitized?" It is 1:00 A.M. and a lecture on how he thought asthma should be dealt with was not of interest to me. I wanted my kid to be relieved of her distress. He ordered an injection, she got it and we waited to see if she would respond. I hadn't fought about it anymore, since I didn't see any other way to make progress and she needed something to help her breathe right away. The pediatrician was reluctant to hospitalize her. "I can't just hospitalize someone; she would have to stay for the whole day. We would have to do a lot of blood tests." What he really meant was he couldn't hospitalize her just because her mother wanted it. After her second injection, Emily was much better. I leaned down to hug her and said, "You're being a real trooper." "That's enough compliments for now," she said, ever-articulate. The decision was made not to hospitalize her, so my brother and I headed for the Yonkers Holiday Inn. Miraculously, the side effects never occurred.

The doctors, for all their obnoxious attitudes, had followed standard protocol for the treatment of asthma. As far as they were concerned, I was a crazy woman off the street, hysterical, and with a hysterical child. I don't know that I would have had much more luck in dealing with anyone, my sister-in-law's pediatrician or anybody else. It's difficult to talk anyone into skipping standard protocol for the treatment of asthma, and that's the dilemma of being away from home. As we arrived at the Holiday Inn, I seriously considered giving up traveling forever.

My brother left us and Emily and I quickly went to sleep. But at 4:30 A.M. she woke again, this time in severe distress and panicky. At this point, the difference between hyperventilation, panic, and asthma doesn't matter. I spent half an hour trying to get her to breathe calmly, but again the inhale to exhale ratio was reversed and her breathing was shallow, rapid and out of control. The interval gave me time to think. I considered going to Montefiore Hospital, which Emily's pediatrician had suggested in case of emergency. Now I was sorry I hadn't followed his advice. But the fact was, I had gotten her away from the cats, the injections were now part of a pattern lasting four hours and she wasn't having side effects. We would be going back to Amherst soon. I might as well go back and get another adrenalin shot. I called my sister-in-law, just to touch base with the world of the sane, and then called the cab company. We arrived in a taxi at 5:30 A.M. The nurse who had been there the whole time stared at us sadly as we came in. Emily went to the bed she had been on before. Her tears fell on the floor as she told the nurse that she could never go back to her uncle's house to play with the dog. The intern looked sympathetic. I wasn't angry or interested in proving that I had been right. At this point I felt as if I were sleepwalking, going through the motions

I had gone through before. She got the shot and they didn't record it. We were not billed for that visit but the other two visits came to $156.00. The motel room was $62.00.

I had asked the taxi to wait outside. She vomited on the sidewalk and we got back in the cab for another $5.00 ride across Yonkers as the sun began to rise over New York. Emily said, "This is a big cab, Mom." I said, "Yeah, well, you probably wouldn't get to ride in a big yellow cab with jump seats unless we were doing this, so let's think of it that way." Back at the Holiday Inn, I called my brother to let him know we were back and called the bus station to find out when we could get a bus. So far I'd had three hours of sleep. I was on automatic pilot. I'm glad my kid hadn't vomited in the back seat of the cab, I thought to myself, but frankly, I didn't care.

I fell asleep and slept for a couple of hours. At 10:30 A.M. I called my brother and said, "Things are better, but we'll have to move fast to catch the 12:30 P.M. bus." My brother picked us up and we drove to his house. Emily waited in the car while I ran in and threw everything in suitcases. My sister-in-law, as always, had the turkey sandwiches and celery sticks and ginger ale packed for us and my brother took a picture of Emily with her beloved friend Peaches, the golden retriever. We all piled into the car and headed for the George Washington Bridge Bus Terminal. When we got there, found a parking space and the ticket window, they said, "Sorry, that bus is filled. That's the express bus, you know."

Through all this, Adrianne had been a real saint. She spent the morning helping my sister-in-law with the baby and getting things organized. I hadn't seen her for twelve hours; she basically got crossed out of the picture. While we waited for the bus, I tried to spend some time talking to her with one eye on Emily. My brother and I discussed what should happen if Emily had trouble on the way home. If things got real bad on the bus, I could ask the bus driver to take me to the police and they would get me to a hospital. At this point I didn't care who got inconvenienced. The whole world could stop while I got the treatment I needed for my kid.

The bus ride back was not bad: five hours on the local route, eating turkey sandwiches. I got several cans of soda into Emily and she actually ate some bits of turkey, to my surprise. We got back and it was 7:00 P.M. before everyone was settled at home. I managed to get a little more food into Emily before the post-asthma-attack complaining session began. She had behaved like a soldier through the worst of it, but safe at home, she began to whine and cling. There is a closeness between mother and child in a severe illness that's like infancy; so much attention must be paid to the child's body that long periods of time are spent in close quarters. Then suddenly it's over. Emily wasn't sure she was ready. I was totally exhausted. Adrianne was edgy, and Emily wanted to sit on my lap. But this was part of the deal. Somehow we got through the evening and Emily went to bed and slept well.

The next day it was hard to tell she had had an asthma episode. Allergic reactions come and go quickly. I sent her to a babysitter's and went to work. But Monday night she had a bad time trying to sleep, apparently a delayed reaction to the whole event: three or four nightmares, restless sleeping, waking up and talking in her sleep. But that was the end of it, at least for her. I needed about a week of sleep.

Could any of it have been changed? When I talked with Emily's pediatrician, he was disappointed that I hadn't called him from the hospital. I had indeed thought about it but it seemed like a crazy idea. He couldn't drive to Yonkers and I couldn't imagine how it would have made things better to have him talk to the doctors on the phone to tell them how to do their jobs. But in thinking about it more, I realized that he could have talked to them and they might indeed have listened. He could have given them a sense of her history and they might have at least have been able to treat her more effectively. Doctors talk to doctors when they don't talk to civilians—that's the way it is.

EMERGENCY DOCTOR LETTER

I had written a few "Dear Doctor" letters for my patients before the Thanksgiving disaster. Emily's experience provoked me to make it a more regular habit. I am willing to write this letter for any child whose parent has taken the Parents' Asthma Course. My secretary types it up after I fill in the blanks. The form and Emily's completed letter are on the following pages.

The best way to deal with an emergency room is to stay away from it. Emergency rooms often do an excellent job of taking care of very sick people. They do not do as well in caring for patients who are moderately ill. One often has to wait a long time for service because people with critical injuries or illness are taken first (as they should be). Follow-up arrangements and advice are often inadequate. Should you feel your child did not receive proper care in an emergency room, you may want to speak with the hospital's "patient representative." If you know how to take care of your child's asthma, you may never have to use an emergency room.

If your child does require emergency care by someone other than your usual physician, you should be able to give her detailed information so that the care for your child can be individualized. A copy of the Asthma Record and the Emergency Room Doctor Letter will provide this necessary information. Emily went back to New York for Thanksgiving in 1982. Her mother and I did everything we could to prepare for the visit. She and her family stayed at a friend's house, rather than living with her uncle's family and the cat. Before her visit she started using her metaproterenol inhaler every four hours. She began taking cromolyn and prednisone one day before the visit began. The three-day visit was peaceful; Emily didn't show a hint of asthma.

Emergency Doctor Letter

Dear Dr.

_____ has asthma.

____ His/her mother/father has taken a four-hour course on asthma for parents. He/She has a good understanding of asthma and the home management needed to control it.

____ He/She uses an adrenergic inhaler, up to four double whiffs a day.

____ His/Her attacks come on quickly and he/she sometimes breathes too quickly to use the inhaler.

____ He/She takes _____ by nebulizer, ____ cc in 2.5 cc saline every four hours when he/she can not use an inhaler.

____ In an emergency his/her usual dose is ____ cc of _____ (__ percent solution) in ____ cc of saline, given every thirty minutes, up to three times.

____ He/She takes theophylline as _____,
____ mg every ____ hours. This amounts to ____ mg/kg/day.

____ His/Her last theophylline level on this dose was ____ mcg/ml on
_____.

____ He/She has received prednisone on ____ occasions in the past year.

____ Early introduction of prednisone in a dose of ____ mg/day has shortened his/her attacks. I usually prescribe for three to seven days.

____ He/She takes cromolyn by (nebulizer, inhaler, Spinhaler) ____ times a day.

____ His/Her last peak flow was _____ liters/minute on ____.

If you have any questions, please call me or my associates at (413) 253-XXXX at any hour of the day or night. Our office is open six days a week and five nights a week; the answering service can reach us at other times. Please make it clear to the answering service that you are a physician and wish to speak to one of the pediatricians.

Sincerely,

_____, M.D.

LETTER FOR EMILY

January 1988

Dear Doctor:

Emily Hall has been treated for chronic asthma of moderate severity since 1979. She was hospitalized overnight for treatment in 1981 and readmitted for two nights in 1986. Her mother has taken a four-hour course on asthma for parents. She has a good understanding of asthma and the home management needed to control it.

Emily takes albuterol, cromolyn, triamcinolone, and ipratropium by metered-dose inhaler, three times a day. Her best peak flow before taking albuterol is 450 liters per minute measured with a Mini-Wright peak flow meter. A drop of greater than twenty percent in her peak flow indicates that she is developing an asthma episode.

Her attacks come on quickly and she sometimes breathes too fast to use the inhaler. In this situation, she will benefit from albuterol by nebulizer, 1.0 cc of a 0.5 percent solution in 2.5 cc saline. This can be followed by two additional doses of albuterol, driven by oxygen, 0.3 cc at thirty minute intervals. She has become over-active, angry, and scared following adrenalin. Inhalation treatment avoids these side effects. A short burst of prednisone, 60 mg per day for three to seven days has shortened her flares.

If you have any questions, please call me or one of my pediatric associates at (413) 253-XXXX at any hour of the day or night. Our office is open six days a week and five nights a week; the answering service can reach us at other times. Please make it clear to the answering service that you are a physician and wish to speak with one of the pediatricians.

Sincerely,

Thomas F. Plaut, M.D.

Monica: The California Trip

■

CELINE CYRAN

In the winter of 1981-82 thirteen-year-old Monica was diagnosed as having asthma. At first I panicked and thought, not that too. One-and-a-half years ago she was diagnosed with scoliosis. Isn't that bad enough? Now that we have that under control, why this? I started thinking about my brother when he was young and the asthma attacks he had.

Monica was planning on spending the summer in California with my sister, Marielle. I wondered if this would change her plans. She had been looking forward to the trip for a long time, but how could I send her 3,000 miles away for someone else to take care of her when I didn't understand what was happening to her myself?

We weathered her first episode with the pediatrician's guidance and reassurance that asthma can be controlled. I started reading all the material he recommended and slowly began to understand what was happening to Monica.

A few months later, Monica had another episode. Naturally my first reaction was to panic again, but I called the doctor and again we got through it all right. In the meantime, my sister was trying to confirm all the plans for Monica to fly out to California. I still didn't feel comfortable with all of this. I knew I needed to learn more so I could cope with Monica's trip.

Our pediatrcian had scheduled a four-hour course for parents of children who have asthma. The sessions that he and his partner held were very productive. It was reassuring to hear the concerns of other parents and to share my feelings with them.

The pediatrician recommended using a stethoscope to learn how to pick up problems with breathing early. Then medication could be given in the beginning stages. The huffer (peak flow meter) was also recommended as a tool to help make decisions about medication. Right away my thoughts were on Monica's trip to California. If I bought the huffer, Monica could monitor her own breathing. After all, I thought, she's almost 14 years old. I was starting to feel better.

After a lengthy consultation with the pediatrician who reassured me that everything would be fine, Monica left with instructions for the care of her asthma. She brought my sister an explanation from the doctor about her asthma, an explanation of medication side effects and a plan for handling any unusual problem. She also had necessary phone numbers, a letter from the pediatrician to an emergency room physician, and my permission releasing responsibility to my sister for emergency room treatment. Naturally I felt much better about everything.

By the time Monica boarded the plane, I felt confident that if an attack occurred:

- Monica could start treating herself.
- If Monica didn't panic, my sister wouldn't panic.
- My sister would be reassured that Monica knew how to take care of herself and could always read the material I sent her.
- They had all the necessary forms and information they would need in case of an emergency.
- I had covered all bases.

When Monica handed my sister the information folder, my sister reacted and said, "What's all this?" Monica replied, "You'd do the same if it was your daughter."

LETTER TO SISTER

Marielle,

Thanks for taking Monica for such a long time this summer. This should be quite an experience for her.

I hope I've sent the information you need as far as Monica's asthma is concerned. I hope it doesn't scare you away. With luck, you won't need any of this. I really hope so; it took me a while to understand what was happening.

There are a few environmental factors that will trigger asthma: house dust (can't get away from), mold, and cigarette smoke. When, and if, she's having difficulty breathing, she should stay away from smoke.

I've enclosed a permission release form for emergency use. (Hope you won't have to use it.)

Monica knows how to use her medicine; she should also know when she needs it. If she uses her huffer to monitor her breathing, she'll be all set.

About a week before she comes back, you can check with the airline to reserve a seat for her in the non-smoking section. Also, she likes window seats.

Enough instructions. Have a good summer.

Lots of Love, Celine

INSTRUCTIONS FOR TREATING
MONICA'S ASTHMA EPISODES

Monica is being treated for asthma. It is of mild severity.

An episode usually comes on after exercise or with an infection.

When she starts to wheeze, she should take Theo-Dur, one-half of a 300 mg tablet, every twelve hours. It should be continued for one day after the wheezing stops.

She should use her inhaler one double whiff every four hours while awake for the first day and then up to four times a day if still wheezing.

If she is not greatly improved after 24 hours of treatment, please contact one of our pediatricians at 413-253-XXXX.

While taking medication for an asthma attack, she should drink at least 64 ounces of liquid a day.

The metaproterenol inhaler should be used fifteen minutes before strenuous exercise to prevent wheezing. The effect usually lasts four hours.

Please check the handouts for side effects of medication.

Call me if you have any questions.

Amy: Vacation Report

■

LYNN LOVELL

Our trip to Florida was interesting, to say the least. We were indeed wise to cart all the paraphenalia and your emergency doctor letter down with us. Yes, Amy had an asthma attack. I knew she would because her peak flow started dropping gradually a few days before the trip. I increased her Bubble treatments (with an inhaled adrenergic drug) but with the climate change and high pollen count Amy went into a moderate-severe episode within three days. She started breathing twice as fast as usual, took longer to breathe out, and couldn't get her peak flow to register at all. Her fever went up to 103.6 degrees and she vomited once.

I didn't have to take her to the hospital because I got her to a good doctor who O.K.d the prednisone treatment. Though it was pretty touch and go, I sensed that she had enough meds in her to weigh the odds in her favor. I was impressed with the doctor. I'm pleased to report that the day-to-day charts you have me fill out earned me instant respect.

Our visit turned out nicely after all. My mother had no idea what I had been going through in dealing with Amy's asthma. Now that she's seen it first hand she understands the situation a lot better. My parents willingly gave me the money to complete payments for the nebulizer. That and the peak flow meter are the best items yet. Amy is doing fine now—no symptoms and still using theophylline twice a day. Thanks for your help and especially your support as I develop my ability to manage Amy's asthma.

7

How to Improve Your Child's Care

How to Choose a Doctor

A child with asthma has a much better chance at leading a normal life when asthma is brought under control through preventive measures. Early intervention can prevent an episode from getting out of control. Only the parents can make the hour to hour observations which will lead to early treatment. Fortunately, many doctors are becoming more comfortable about accepting parents as partners in the treatment of asthma.

What should you look for when choosing a doctor for your child with asthma? There are two main issues to deal with. First, does the doctor know about asthma? Second, will the doctor help you to learn to manage your child's asthma at home? You can use the following three criteria as a test of minimum acceptable competence for your child's asthma doctor.

Does the doctor give written instructions when prescribing medications? This reduces the possibility of misunderstandings and errors in treatment.

Does the office staff teach your child how to use any prescribed device (inhaler, holding-chamber, nebulizer) and monitor your child's technique? Even if they are taught perfectly, many children make mistakes and don't get the full benefit of a device unless they are checked regularly.

Does the doctor or staff measure peak expiratory flow rate in the office to assess your child's status at each visit? The peak flow information is essential for adjusting medications properly.

If your answer to these three questions is yes you are going to a doctor you can consider working with.

Minimum Criteria for Asthma Doctor

- Gives written instructions

- Teaches and monitors use of devices

- Measures peak flow each visit

Now you need to decide how well the physician's attitude toward home management fits in with yours. Please remember, no matter how good the doctor, you have the primary responsibility for your child's care. A good doctor will teach you how to care for your child's asthma within certain well-defined limits.

In order to assist parents to manage asthma at home properly, a physician has to have comprehensive knowledge of asthma and the drugs used to treat it, the skill to instruct and monitor parents in the use of a peak flow meter and new medication, and an attitude that recognizes the parents as the primary managers of their child's asthma. Finally, the physician must also support parents as they learn about asthma, must be readily accessible, and must treat parents as intelligent, concerned partners in the care of their child's asthma.

Which doctor can help you care for your child with asthma? The physician's specialty is not nearly as important as his or her interest in asthma. An interested pediatrician can help you care for most children with asthma without help. He or she will request a consultation from an allergist or a pulmonologist (lung specialist) to assist in the care of those children who have more severe or complicated problems.

HOW OFTEN SHOULD YOU SEE THE DOCTOR?

How often should a child be seen for review of his or her asthma status and treatment planning? The child with very mild asthma which is controlled by the use of one drug and who never misses school because of asthma should be seen once a year for review of treatment plan, treatment technique, to uncover hidden symptoms of asthma, and to bring parents up to date on improvements in treatment for asthma.

Any child who has missed school or limited activity due to asthma should have a thorough review at least every six months. Any child who is taking three or more drugs for asthma should have a thorough review at least every four months.

During the period in which parents are learning to manage asthma and we are determining the proper treatment plan, we may see them once a month or even more often. Unscheduled urgent visits do not substitute for a planned review. Only the basic aspects of asthma management can be learned at the time of an asthma flare. Fine tuning of the treatment plan must take place at a more relaxed time.

SEEKING A CONSULTATION

Even when parents have had a good experience and work well with their child's physician, they may want a second opinion on some prescribed course of action. This is accepted medical practice, and parents should not feel at all uncomfortable in asking for a consultation.

Under what circumstances should you request a consultation with another doctor?

If your child limits his or her activity or misses school because of asthma, you should review the situation with your regular doctor or seek a second opinion.

If your child has to go to the emergency room for care more than once, the asthma is probably not well-controlled. Either you don't know how to take care of it or your child's asthma is not being treated adequately. You should review the situation with your doctor or seek another opinion.

If your child is hospitalized more than once for asthma you should obtain a consultation in order to review overall treatment.

If your physician suggests that your child limit his or her activities because of asthma, it would be wise to seek a second opinion. Almost all children with asthma can participate in any sport if they are receiving proper care—unless they are in the middle of an asthma flare.

Consultation needed if

- child limits activity

- emergency treatment more than once

- hospitalized more than once

- doctor says to limit activity

In order to get maximum benefit from a consultation with an asthma specialist I suggest you prepare in the following manner. Read this book completely and make sure you can answer every question on the asthma quiz on page 68. Fill out the asthma consultation form on page 207. Type out a narrative of your child's asthma history. Ask your regular doctor to provide a summary of your child's asthma problem. Bring any additional information that you think is important. The materials you prepare will provide your consultant with a comprehensive view of your child's asthma problem. As a result you will accomplish as much in one consultation as most people accomplish in two or three. Many parents bring their spouse, a relative, or a friend to join them for the consultation. This makes the visit less intimidating. It also marks the creation of an asthma support system.

I suggest that you involve your child's regular physician by asking that he or she provide a clinical summary and suggest a consultant. A competent physician will not be insulted by this request. In fact he or she will want to provide names of consultants who would be particularly skilled to help with your child's care. However, some parents prefer to make all the consultation arrangements on their own. I support their right to do so.

Asthma Consultation Form

Please fill in information. Circle correct answers when you are given a choice. Ignore questions that you can't answer.

What would you like to learn or what changes would you like to see as a result of this consultation?

1. Name:

2. Date of birth:

3. Age at onset of wheezing or chronic cough:

4. Age at diagnosis:

5. Frequency of episodes (an episode is any flare of asthma which requires the patient to modify activity or take medication):

   /year   /month   continuous

6. Number of school days missed in the past twelve months:

7. Triggers:
   respiratory infection   pollutants   cold air
   exercise   allergens   other

8. Early clues: cough   watery eyes
                  sneeze   behavior change
                  scratchy throat

9. Year, month and duration of each hospitalization for respiratory problems with diagnosis of bronchiolitis, bronchitis, pneumonia, or asthma:

10. Number of emergency room visits in the past twelve months:

11. Name three changes in the windpipe caused by asthma:

12. What are the four most important things to monitor during an asthma episode?

13. Medications taken at present time (dose and frequency):

    adrenergic

    theophylline

    cromolyn

    prednisone

    antibiotic

    immunotherapy (allergy shots)

14. Name one action of each medication your child takes:

15. Does child have eczema, rhinitis, sinusitis, hives, gastric reflux?

16. Family history:
    Asthma?   Who?
    Hay Fever?   Who?
    Eczema?   Who?

17. Environment:

    Does anyone in the house smoke?

    Heating source: oil   gas   electric   wood   coal   other

    Heat distribution: radiant   hot water   steam   hot air

    Type of cooking: gas   electric   wood   other

    Any pets?

House: age, location, type of construction

Have you:

18. Kept an asthma diary?

19. Read *Children With Asthma: A Manual For Parents*?

20. Attended an asthma education session?

21. Been instructed in environmental control?

22. Been instructed in the use of a

    metered-dose inhaler?

    holding chamber (InspirEase, INHAL-AID, paper tube, AeroChamber)?

    peak flow meter?

    compressor powered nebulizer?

    Spinhaler?

23. Consulted a physician other than your regular doctor regarding asthma?

I Wish Doctors Would

Parents in the asthma group completed the sentence, "When dealing with parents of children who have asthma I wish doctors would . . ." as follows:

- be as clear and open as possible about all aspects—how to deal with attacks, medication, what's really happening, danger—all the topics dealt with in this workshop.
- tell the parent how long to keep giving these high doses of medication before cutting back.
- teach how to prevent attacks.

- explain what else goes on besides the wheeze.
- be completely honest—but not use scare tactics.
- prescribe and stipulate the precise medication but give the boundaries within which I can make decisions on my own.
- have told me sooner that it was asthma I was dealing with instead of a respiratory infection.
- continue just the way they have been.
- assume that the parent is a reasonably intelligent individual who knows her child in a way the doctor doesn't—and that they can learn from each other how best to treat the child.
- explain precautions before an episode and remedies during and after.
- tell us more.
- be straightforward.
- be better informed.
- encourage all concerned to vent their fears.
- provide lots of information.
- not make me feel that I brought the child in for nothing.
- put articles in newspapers.
- explain everything more.
- if they don't know about asthma—send the patient to a doctor who does.

My New Doctor Listens

■

CATHLEEN HENNING, FLORIDA

The day I read your book was truly a day of awakening for me. I realized that it was totally unnecessary for my son to be receiving a shot of adrenalin as the only conclusion to each and every attack he had. My three-year-old child was taking 400 mg of theophylline a day and bouncing off the walls from its effects. We made seemingly endless trips to the six different on-call pediatricians (my son has weekend asthma) to enable him to breathe normally.

The pediatricians were treating the asthma episodically and telling me to consult the allergist if I needed anything further. The allergist told me to take Douglas, my son, to the pediatricians for routine treatments. By the time I found your book, I was ready to move to Phoenix, the beaches, or to get an M.D. degree so that I could treat him myself! The day I arrived at the allergist's office, your book in hand, asking to discuss whether Douglas would benefit from cromolyn, I was treated as a necessary evil who had to be dealt with and forgotten. He gave us a prescription for cromolyn, but when I tried to explain to him what the INHAL-AID was and that I thought it would be better for Douglas than a small-volume holding chamber, he told me he had never heard of it, that he did not want to see your book, and that there was no need for me to be asking about albuterol, steroids, or any other medications. A well-informed mother was a threat to this man. Yet, somehow, I no longer cared. I trusted my new knowledge enough to know that I wanted to play an active role in Douglas' care. My next choice of allergist would be one who respected my knowledge of my child's needs as well as my knowledge of asthma, and my desire to prevent the attacks rather than treat them episodically.

At our first visit with the new allergist, he asked me to review Douglas' medical history and treatment. He asked questions and *listened* to my answers *and* opinions. He immediately demonstrated and prescribed the INHAL-AID! I asked for an adrenergic inhaler to replace the albuterol liquid that made Douglas irritable and sleepless during the attacks. He agreed, and prescribed an inhaler with a liquid adrenergic as a backup. I told him that cromolyn had maintained Douglas without an attack for the previous five months, and he agreed that we should continue with it and use theophylline only as needed. Finally, when I asked him if he would be interested in reading *Children With Asthma: A Manual For Parents,* and explained your concept of teaching parents to manage asthma at home, he borrowed the book, read it, ordered his own copy, and now recommends it to parents. When I expressed an interest in starting a support group, he provided me with literature from the Allergy and Asthma Foundation of America and now has provided referrals to our group.

I left that first visit with a written plan for treatment that I knew would work for my son, and a tremendous sense of relief. What a difference it made to have the support and confidence of a doctor who was more concerned with my child's well-being than with his own insecurities about who was going to control my child's care.

In the last ten months, through the use of a well-established plan of preventive maintenance and early intervention, we have had only two episodes that actually reached "attack" proportions. Only once did I need to call the doctor, at which point we decided on an increased dose of medication. That was it. It worked. No expensive and painful trip to the emergency room. NO SHOT!

Douglas is nearly five now, playing soccer, swimming—a normal, healthy child with occasional flares of asthma, and I can't even remember his last shot of adrenalin!

Together with Pam Greenman, I started a support group in the Jacksonville area. Our group is now an active, educational and support network of thirteen families and is still growing. We appreciate all the literature you have sent us and especially the video tape. We have shown it at our meetings and all agree that it is like seeing the book come to life!

I Can Talk With My Doctor
■

KRISTINE URAVICH, IDAHO

Julie had been coughing for three months following a suspected case of pneumonia in January. She was only two-and-a half then and could not describe how she was feeling. She looked healthy and her growth continued to be good. But she coughed all the time. She stayed awake at night, propped high on bed pillows and engulfed in the vapor of a cool mist machine. She coughed so hard that tiny blood vessels broke in her cheeks. Our doctor prescribed what seemed to be gallons of metaproterenol syrup, and later what he described as a "powerful drug" (slow-release theophylline) to help open her airways.

Our family doctor gave me lots of explanations: it's a lung irritation, maybe she's allergic to your dog, her lungs were temporarily damaged by the infection. We took her to an allergist for skin patch tests, got rid of our long-time family dog and tried to free our home of housedust.

But, she was still "sick." Late one afternoon in April, during a particularly hard cold, I crawled into Julie's bed to try and help her sleep. Her breathing was labored and fast. I became frightened. Maybe she would stop breathing. Maybe she would die!

Our family doctor was out of town, so I called the allergist in a town forty miles from home. After a brief exam in his office, the doctor handed me a prescription. "What's wrong with her?" I wanted to know. The reply was so matter-of-fact that I was stunned: She was having an asthma attack! I had never heard the word "asthma" used in association with my daughter's health.

That's when I began to learn about asthma. That's when I decided that the day-in/day-out medical care for this child was in my hands. I had to find out about symptoms, medications, and treatment. I needed the information necessary to ask intelligent questions during doctor visits. I would be my child's advocate in the doctor's office.

Through an article on asthma in "American Baby" magazine, I learned about *Children with Asthma: A Manual For Parents*. I read it through the day it arrived in the mail and went to the doctor's office with a barrage of questions. Our family doctor was at first surprised by some of them. He had assumed that I would prefer to give theophylline at breakfast and supper rather than every twelve hours as recommended. I think he should have asked me. He didn't realize that I would gladly inconvenience myself to help my child to breathe better.

When I inquired about the advantages that I would gain by delivering medicine for Julie with a compressor-driven nebulizer, he told me he thought it was too expensive and too complicated for me to manage. After some discussion, he agreed to let me make the decision.

After that, things began to go our way. We purchased a compressor-driven nebulizer for use at home. It is simple to operate and was paid for primarily by our insurance coverage. We got a firm grip on asthma through a good medication routine. Most importantly, I've learned that professional medical treatment is a service that requires intelligent consideration by the patient as a consumer. In order to deal effectively with my physician, I must be informed. I need to be able to describe symptoms in terms the doctor understands and know the whys and hows of drugs so we can use them properly and effectively. Using my physician as a "consultant" I have accepted the responsibility of managing Julie's asthma until she is old enough to take it on herself.

Admission to the Hospital

Doctors' attitudes toward hospitalization for asthma vary greatly. This will be an important factor in your choice of a physician for your child. If your doctor is skilled as a consultant in home treatment, hospitalization for asthma should be a rare event. However, admission is necessary if a child is having serious difficulty with breathing which cannot be improved by aggressive treatment in the office or emergency room. The child with moderate breathing difficulty may also require admission if his or her situation is deteriorating in spite of aggressive treatment.

Under what circumstances should a child be admitted to a hospital? Admission is necessary if essential observation and treatment cannot be provided in the home, office, or emergency room. The heart rate, blood pressure, and breathing status should be closely monitored. Sometimes medications must be given in large doses. When nebulized adrenergics are needed more often than every four hours, they are often given with oxygen. This intensive observation and treatment cannot be done at home.

Other factors to be considered in making a decision to hospitalize are:

- the availability of physician coverage. This often declines drastically at nighttime or on weekends.
- availability of nursing staff and proper equipment in the outpatient facility.

- the physician's experience in supervising the care of a moderately ill child with asthma by phone.
- the parents' knowledge of asthma and the medications used to treat it.
- the parents' skill in use of various devices such as a compressor-driven nebulizer and the peak flow meter to manage asthma.
- availability of telephone and transportation.
- other demands on the parents.

If a parent appears in the emergency room with a child having an asthma episode, it means to me that the parents have exhausted their resources to assess and treat asthma at home. Perhaps the family has no regular physician or the regular physician was not available to assist in the care of their child.

If a doctor recommends admission to the hospital for your child who is having a serious asthma flare, this is not the time to assert independence. You can describe your resources to handle asthma at home but don't fight the admission. The best way to avoid an admission is to work out a written plan in advance with your physician. If you learn how to monitor the four signs of asthma trouble, the peak flow rate, and how to start treatment early, hospitalization can usually be avoided.

Some of our patients who are admitted to the hospital had not been treated previously for asthma. Since they had no experience with asthma, these parents were unable to recognize that their child had a breathing problem until it had progressed to the point where we could not remedy it in our office.

Cooperating physicians in the national Asthma Project were asked to analyze the records of patients they admitted to the hospital. In almost every case they felt the admission could not have been avoided at the time the patient was seen. However, a future admission for asthma might be avoided if

- a piece of equipment (a peak flow meter, a compressor-driven nebulizer) were available to the patient.
- medications were started earlier.
- steroids were started earlier.
- the parents' understanding of asthma were improved.
- a complete written plan were available for the parents.

The hospital is a good place to learn about asthma by reading, watching video tapes, and discussing questions and concerns with nurses, respiratory therapists, and doctors. You should be able to find a copy of *Teaching Myself About Asthma* and *Luke Has Asthma, Too* on the pediatric ward. Each of the books will be fun and educational to read with your child. Many hospitals have video tapes about asthma which you can watch at your child's beside. Most pediatric nurses have cared for many children with asthma. They should be able to answer many of your questions. Respiratory therapists are particularly helpful in teaching parents how to use a peak flow meter and how to use and clean a compressor-driven nebulizer and holding chamber.

If parents learn how to use a compressor-driven nebulizer in the hospital, they can use this machine to give their child medication at home. We reduce the length of hospitalizations by sending patients home using compressor-driven nebulizer treatment before their symptoms have cleared completely. Obviously, this can only be done if careful followup can be arranged. We usually see patients within twenty-four to forty-eight hours after discharge from the hospital to review their status.

All in all, the hospital admission should be a good learning experience. If you learn enough about asthma and its treatment, a second admission will rarely be necessary.

Epilogue

A few years have gone by since parents spoke in earlier pages about their children's asthma. We close with a more recent look at these children and then answer some frequently asked questions.

Parents' expectations of these seven children are high. They anticipate that each will be able to participate in all activities no matter how strenuous. These parents have accepted a monitoring routine and a medication plan, but they have accepted asthma symptoms only on a very temporary basis. The children have high expectations of themselves. They know that asthma is not an excuse to miss school or to do less than their peers. They expect to participate fully in all activities.

We doctors also have high expectations. We predict that emergencies will rarely arise since parents will do an excellent job of monitoring and caring for their children.

Casey

■

CAROLINE TROPP

We moved to New Hampshire when Casey was three years old. I was nervous about Casey's asthma because we now lived 150 miles from our old pediatrician. Casey's new doctor was very helpful and respected me and my knowledge about Casey's asthma. When he said that I know enough to judge Casey's medication needs, I got my confidence back.

The first year was very difficult. I was only working part time and money was very tight. Casey's medicine was so expensive. He was supposed to take cromolyn four times a day, an adrenergic drug four times a day, and theophylline three times a day. The bill for these medicines came to fifteen dollars per week.

I couldn't afford to give the medicine as often as I should have. I figured that once my medical insurance went through it would take care of his medication bills. However, the insurance company denied coverage for Casey because of his asthma! I was mortified and mad. How could I afford to buy the medication for my son? There had to be a way to get help. I applied for Medicaid just to cover Casey's bills. They turned me down because I made $92.50 working twenty hours per week. This was five dollars over the eligibility limit.

I kept looking for ways to get help. Finally a social worker told me that the Handicapped Children's Program in the Department of Human Services would pay for medication for kids with asthma. I never considered Casey to be handicapped but without proper medication I guess he would be. They accepted my application and finally he got the medicines he needed.

A good friend of ours who has asthma owns a compressor-driven nebulizer. We used it at his house any time Casey had a severe attack day or night. It really worked well. When our old doctor heard about it, he sent us a nebulizer so we could use it at home on a regular basis.

It's been a tough road. I now have two jobs and sometimes I feel guilty because I haven't regulated Casey's treatment as well as I should have. My money problem has now changed to a time problem. Also, did you ever try to sit a very active five-year-old boy down to use a nebulizer for ten minutes three times a day? That's a task in itself.

We see the doctor in Amherst about every four months to review Casey's progress. He has not been in a hospital emergency room since we got his asthma under control two years ago. I think we are doing well. However, Casey still has trouble coughing at night and also gets flares in the cold weather. Our doctor says Casey should be able to do anything he wants without having asthma symptoms. Why not? Why can't my son be fully active? I guess I had the feeling that it would never happen but why underestimate what we can do? Now my goal is to get rid of all Casey's symptoms.

Ryan

■

DANA PARKER

November 1981 seems ages ago. The date of Ryan's first asthma flare is only a scary memory. Things are sedate now by comparison. Ryan often uses an albuterol inhaler before exercise to prevent symptoms. He took long-acting theophylline for three flares in the past year. Two of them lasted a few days, the third a few weeks.

Ryan is physically growing out of the acute, serious, and frequent episodes that marked his fourth year. We are more alert to his particular triggers. They include any form of cut grass or hay, any cold or flu in the winter months, and up until recently, any form of animal dander. Ryan is able to judge how close he dare go to those things, and self-manages well. With regard to the new family cat, Ryan showed great patience. He measured his distances and doses of the cat cautiously until after about eight weeks he showed little or no sign of reaction to the cat. Our doctor disapproves. He says Ryan may become allergic to the cat.

Ryan started preschool when he was four years old. The school was apprehensive, both because of his history of severe asthma episodes and also because he was overactive and hard to interest for very long when taking his standard dose of theophylline. These qualities persisted when he entered kindergarten. A very supportive school staff and school nurse helped him greatly with his medicines and in attending to the tasks of school.

By first grade his need for daily theophylline decreased dramatically. His inhaler took care of most symptoms. At the same time he became very much attuned to the academic aspects of first grade. He has done extremely well in school and is now in the second grade.

Ryan understands his asthma very well. At the same time, he has come to dislike his condition. When he is wheezing and coughing he gets sad and often angry. But we feel a sense of progress because since his first episode he has improved steadily. His symptoms are milder and are easier to relieve each year.

Matthew

■

JEAMIE DUFFY

The second half of Matthew's story is very different from the first. The first chapter left off when Matthew was about seven years old and just out of the hospital from an asthma attack. He is now eleven and no longer on daily medication. He is still a happy, outgoing, fun-loving individual and, thankfully, one who no longer has severe asthma. He still has intermittent trouble and still must take medicine, but not on a daily basis. I never thought it would happen.

The course of Matthew's asthma did not really change between age seven and ten. Throughout those years he took a wide variety of medications and continued to have trouble quite frequently. But his health was no longer the focal point in any of our lives. He took part in baseball, basketball, and football; his asthma was never an issue. Only when necessary did we even discuss it (for example, when visiting a friend who had an animal), and then only as much as required.

When Matthew was nine, we moved from Amherst to Rochester, Minnesota. I knew it would be difficult to adjust to a new medical environment and I did not look forward to finding a doctor who would accept our involvement in the management of Matthew's health. To convince the doctor that I knew what I was talking about, I brought a copy of *Children with Asthma* and quickly pointed out my chapter. I was expecting resistance. I received none. The doctor was more than willing to accept my knowledge and interest concerning Matthew's health.

Things went on unremarkably until the spring when Matthew was ten. He began his usual symptoms of having trouble. Unfortunately, we ignored them. We had been lulled into a false sense of security. Because of this, we did not intervene quickly enough. We had actually forgotten how to handle an asthma attack. Because of this delay, Matthew got into more trouble than was necessary and had to be hospitalized. That was his first hospitalization in three years. It was less traumatic than I expected and after three days, Matthew was back to his old self.

About six months ago, Joe and I decided that it was about time Matt took responsibility for his medication. He was familiar with what he needed and could handle all aspects himself. As one would expect from an eleven year old, he forgot most of the time. Joe and I reasoned that he would discover the consequences of not taking his medicine (he would wheeze) and then remember to take what he needed. Were we fooled! He never wheezed. So, of course, he did not take his medicine. After talking to his doctor, we decided to give "no medicine" a try. After six months, all is still going well. We are taking this experiment one day at a time, or should I say one season at a time.

The only sad aspect to Matthew's current health is with regard to animals. As his asthma got better, his desire for a dog got stronger. About a year ago, after much debate, we decided to give a family dog a try. A friend of mine raises dogs and I explained the situation to her. I asked if we could take one of her puppies on a trial basis. She agreed and we brought Max home. We had told Matthew the conditions under which we got the dog and hoped he would understand. After only a few hours, we all had watery eyes and both Joe and Matthew started to wheeze. Somehow I was not surprised. We gave the dog back the next morning. I asked Matthew if he wished he had never tried and he answered that one day with a dog was better than nothing.

People who have only known Matthew since we moved here do not know him as "an asthmatic," only as the great kid he is. When they hear some of the stories about his early years, they can't believe them. I feel fortunate that who Matthew really is no longer has anything to do with his health.

Nathan
∎

MARILYN SANSOUCI

In the past two years Nathan has had a tremendous improvement in his health. I am grateful for the knowledge I gained on how to deal with asthma and for the parents who shared their experiences on how to cope with asthma. It is nice to know that others have dealt with this problem. My husband David gives me a lot of support and help.

Nathan now has asthma episodes twice a year. He has one in the spring and one in the late fall. That is a real improvement from having an episode every other month. Nathan still takes a long-acting theophylline preparation three times a day. Recently he had an attack and we started giving metaproterenol by nebulizer four to six times a day. He also took predisone twice a day for a week. After a couple days of treatment Nathan was fine and as playful and active as ever.

Nathan loves to ride his bike and play baseball with his three older brothers. He is excited about starting kindergarten this fall. I'm so happy with Nathan's progress. It is a relief not to be frantic and upset with worry if he does have an asthma episode. I believe the key to overcoming the problem of asthma is to detect it early and to give the child proper treatment.

Each child has different symptoms. In Nathan's case he will get itchy, usually behind his ears and on his chest, and he might be cranky for a couple of days. Then he will start symptoms of a cold and he'll start wheezing. Now that Nathan is getting older he knows when he starts to have trouble and he will come to me and ask for a nebulizer treatment.

Asthma is a problem, but as long as we know enough to treat it properly, we can go on and live normal happy lives. I am going to have my fifth baby this September. People have asked me, "Well, aren't you worried about your new baby having asthma?" Of course I hope and pray that this new baby will not have asthma. But I am not too worried because my husband and I know how to deal with it.

Josh

■

HARRIET GOODWIN

Josh is now in tenth grade. Among his main interests at the moment is karate, which he has been studying for the past three years. He has held a blue belt for a while now and is hoping to achieve a black belt before he graduates from high school. Skateboarding has pushed breakdancing out of the picture recently, and Josh has just bought himself a motor scooter with some of the money he has earned working with his father. He shows a certain disdain for his ten-speed, but he's keeping his dirt bike.

Asthma? Oh yes, that's still a part of Josh's life, but it is no longer the way in which he identifies himself to others.

About five years ago Josh was hospitalized and we both learned a great deal from that experience. By living through it I lost my terror of "going to the hospital" as a worst-case scenario. Now I look at the hospital as a non-threatening place where they have all the same medicines that we do at home, but also have a few more, some extra gadgets to dispense them with, and nurses who can make hour to hour observations. Although we have conquered our fear of hospitalization, it does enlarge my leverage with Josh when he gets careless with his medication routine. Just one reminder of that event convinces him to take his medicine.

Josh does take his medication on his own, except at times of severe distress. Sometimes he has trouble because he has been "careless" about his medication. I tell him what the doctor repeatedly tells me: it's his body, and if he doesn't take care of himself, he will get sick, not me. He has the responsibility to take the medication and limit his physical activities at these rare times. I have to face the fact that I can't yank him off his skateboard—he's going too fast, already out of sight and downtown anyway! Of course, it is hard for a parent to stay on the sidelines. By and large, I do, and for the most part, Josh manages quite well.

Josh has not taken theophylline in the past year. His headaches have decreased dramatically and evening nausea and vomiting is a thing of the past. He is stabilized on a routine of using the cromolyn inhaler three double puffs a day and the albuterol inhaler three to five times a day. He uses the albuterol before sports and sometimes at night. When he ceases to get relief from this routine, Josh uses a short burst of prednisone. This happens two or three times a year. We see the doctor every four months to review asthma care rather than to treat an flare.

Just recently Josh had a brief but major crisis. The triggering complications were flu and an ear infection. Suddenly Josh went from just being sick and feverish to having great difficulty with his breathing. He begged me to take him to the doctor— an unheard-of request from Josh. His peak flow score was down and Josh had retractions. His breathing out took longer than breathing in. I was scared and I was out of practice. I was unsure about how to handle this episode. I started him on prednisone, and managed to track down our doctor for guidance by phone. Over a few hours' time Josh seemed to turn a corner. The next morning he was much better.

Why is it always at night, never during office hours? This time I found out the answer—asthma always gets worse during the night. It's a steady twenty-four hour cycle, for everyone, better in the day, worse at night.

As a result of this crisis we paid a visit to the office. As usual, we learned something new. Our doctor introduced us to the concept of dividing peak flow readings into the green, yellow, and red zones. We used these zones to formulate a written treatment plan. Now that we've established these guides for action I feel like a general with a strategic battle plan almost guaranteed to work.

At this stage of my lengthy experience as an asthma parent, the hardest part for me is helping Josh decide what to do and when to do it during a crisis. The burden of that responsibility seems light when I look back to the pain, guilt, fear, and sadness which I experienced when I first began to realize that I was the parent of a person who has asthma.

Russ

■

RUSSELL T. WALL

I have suffered from asthma for most of my nineteen years. Many a cold winter night I have spent hour upon hour gasping for air in a hospital Emergency Room. I have battled with many bouts of "pneumonia" that left me underweight and demoralized. Every head cold I caught would immediately invade my lungs and spark breathing difficulty. On top of that, I suffered from side effects of the drug, theophylline. I would lose sleep because of the stimulant effect of theophylline. Headaches added more discomfort. I had to choose, either breathe easier and accept the side effects or skip the drug and wind up in the Emergency Room. Some choice. I would always choose to accept the breathing difficulty. It seemed like the safest route.

I oppose any kind of drug-taking and feel that drugs and sports just don't mix. Though I knew I could breathe easier if I took drugs I chose to play without them. Recently I have learned that the theophylline was all right, the doctors were just giving me too much of it.

Four months before I was to leave for Arizona State University I had one of the worst asthma attacks ever. I required Emergency Room treatment three times in one week. This was not good. I was going to be on my own soon and felt a need to get my asthma under control.

I visited a new doctor and started reading about asthma and the medications used to treat it. I was amazed at the number of ways that asthma can be defeated. After some experimenting we figured out that if I reduced my theophylline dose I could get relief without getting headache, nausea, or sleeplessness. I would use albuterol to prevent or treat episodes caused by exercise. A short burst of prednisone could be used if my symptoms didn't clear quickly. He assured me that this plan would hold up, but if it didn't, he was confident we could work out another.

The doctor also introduced me to the peak flow meter. What a device! For the first time I could actually "see" how well I was breathing. At first I thought of it as just another pain in the butt, another waste of time. One of my college roommates saw the peak flow meter and wanted to try it. When others came in to measure their peak flow I started a competition. The person with the highest score would win a prize (usually a hamburger or pizza). Over a period of months, I began equalling and then surpassing kids who didn't have asthma. What a thrill it was to actually see my progression. Due to the peak flow meter, I could see myself getting better and I was elated.

The peak flow meter also allows me to stay off medication because on days when I "see" that I'm breathing well, I simply don't take medication. One day after a couple of sets of tennis, I checked my peak flow and found it was a little under par. I immediately started taking medication and two days later I was back up to my usual mark.

Today I sit here in sunny Arizona and my horrible memories of asthma seem to disappear. I feel stronger and healthier now than at any time in my life. When you get right down to it, asthma is just another opponent. As in any sport, you can defeat asthma with knowledge and practice.

Emily
∎
GAIL HALL

The Thanksgiving Disaster has faded in my memory over the past five years. I'm not sure how I survived that experience. We now regularly visit my brother, and Emily's asthma takes a back seat to the needs of her three cousins, ages five and under. This happy switch in focus is the result of several important changes. In addition to my brother and sister-in-law's tireless efforts to make their house an allergen-free environment, I've developed a new approach and learned to use new tools for dealing with Emily's health. As a result, I no longer think about delaying or cancelling travel plans because of asthma.

One of the most important things I did after the Thanksgiving Disaster was to get more information about Emily's asthma. We learned from allergy tests that she reacted not only to cats but to wool and horse hair. Both were present in quantity in the room we had mistakenly assumed to be a safe haven in my brother's house. He has since ripped out the rugs and old fashioned rug mats which the previous owners had left.

Another important change was in my attitude. On our ill-fated trip, I kept hoping that things would take care of themselves. I assumed that nothing new would happen and that I had seen the worst that allergy-induced asthma could do. In fact, hoping instead of acting on the problem ruined the trip. Nowadays, I start out prepared for the worst and begin treatment at the first sign of trouble. I carry all of Emily's medication in a large travel bag. When she goes on an overnight at a neighbor's, she arrives with emergency instructions, the doctor-to-doctor letter, her albuterol inhaler and her cromolyn inhaler. She also brings the huffer and, if she's going more than 25 miles from home, the nebulizer. It's a bit overwhelming and intrusive, but it beats going to the emergency room.

The huffer (peak flow meter) allows an untrained person, such as the parent who's hosting the overnight, to tell whether Emily is in trouble. When she travels out of town by herself, I enclose a card indicating at which peak flow readings I should be called, she should be brought home, or she should be taken to a hospital and my pediatrician called.

Two summers ago, I sent both of my daughters on a visit to my brother in Chicago. Halfway to the airport I realized that the huffer was still sitting on the kitchen table. When I got home, I sent it off through the Post Office's overnight mail. The trip was a major success. Using the huffer at medication time, my sister-in-law was able to assure herself (and me, when I called) that there were no changes in the way Emily was breathing. After that, I decided I needed a master list of medications and equipment and a central place to keep everything.

The compressor-driven nebulizer is something my pediatrician talked me into. It sat in a closet for six months, Emily's asthma having become a milder and milder condition in the last few years. But finally a cold set in to her chest and her peak flow continued to drop for two days, despite the fact that I had increased medications immediately. I pulled out the nebulizer and had Emily use it while she watched television. (It takes ten minutes or so; distractions are helpful.) Her score went up one hundred points in half an hour, the biggest increase I'd ever seen without injections. Plus, the side effects were minimal. Using the nebulizer meant she missed one day of school that week instead of four. Now I use the nebulizer routinely. If her peak flow doesn't return to normal with an extra whiff of the inhaler, I introduce the nebulizer the same day and check in with the doctor on whether to add other medications.

While I seem to have a lot of asthma "baggage" these days I think about it less. I've left behind a lot of my embarrassment and also the idea that if I prepare less, less will happen. People admire the way my family handles asthma and I enjoy that. Asthma was more of a burden when I had fewer gadgets to carry around.

Common Questions

These questions are organized according to the section headings in chapters two, three, four, and five.

Basic Facts

ATTACKS

Q. What are some other words for an asthma attack?

A. Episode and flare. These words are used interchangeably.

Q. What is an asthma attack?

A. Any episode of asthma which involves worsening of breathing that interrupts on-going activities or requires some procedure, such as resting or taking medicine, to resume normal and comfortable breathing.

Q. How can you predict an asthma episode?

A. Contact with a trigger that has set off an episode in the past makes it likely that one will occur again. A drop in peak flow of more than twenty percent indicates interference with air flow and means that significant symptoms may occur soon.

Q. What is the usual duration of an asthma flare?

A. Flares triggered by exercise may last only two hours. Some episodes triggered by an upper respiratory infection may last for two weeks. Each individual seems to have his own pattern or set of patterns.

Q. How can you tell if a child is having an asthma flare if there is no wheezing, just a bad cough, congestion or a lousy cold?

A. A cold is an upper respiratory infection, caused by a virus that primarily affects the nose, throat and sinuses. Congestion is the stuffiness caused by swelling of the tissues in the nose. Asthma is often triggered by a cold and thus may occur at the same time. Asthma affects the lower respiratory tract. Its symptoms are not cleared by coughing, sneezing or blowing your nose. You can check for asthma by using the peak flow meter. Our motto is, "If it gets better with asthma medicine, it is probably asthma."

Q. Why does a flare sometimes follow a virus infection and other times not?

A. An episode may be set off by a strong trigger or by a combination of weak triggers. A cold plus some pollution will trigger an attack when either one alone may not.

Q. What is acute bronchitis?

A. The term bronchitis refers to an inflammation of the large airways caused by a virus infection.

Q. How often do children get acute bronchitis?

A. Most children who get acute bronchitis never get it again. If it recurs, the diagnosis of asthma should be considered.

TRIGGERS

Q. How hard should I work to keep my child away from things that trigger his/her asthma flares?

A. Your caution should match the seriousness of the problem. If the child gets a severe attack after coming in contact with a cat, you should try to avoid cats. If that is impossible, try pretreatment with an adrenergic drug and/or cromolyn to block an episode. Children who wheeze with exercise should use their inhaler before they start practicing or competing.

Q. How can I learn about triggers?

A. The best way is to keep a careful record of the child's activities during an asthma flare. You will learn quite quickly what situations seem to cause trouble. Standard triggers are viral infections, exercise, irritants, allergens, and mechanical triggers such as coughing, laughing, and yelling.

Q. Can aspirin cause an asthma attack?

A. Aspirin will trigger an attack in one or two percent of children with asthma. This problem is much more common with adults.

ENVIRONMENT

Q. Can heating with a wood stove trigger an asthma episode?

A. Yes, even a tight wood stove draws smoke pollution from outside into the house.

Q. What is the best humidity for the environment of a child with asthma?

A. The mucous membranes of the body function best in clearing irritants at a humidity of 25–40 percent.

ALLERGY AND ALLERGY SHOTS

Q. What allergens should I look out for?

A. If your child starts wheezing after contact with an animal (dog, cat, or pony) you can be quite sure that the child is allergic to that animal's dander.

Q. If I get rid of the cat and the house dust, will my child's asthma improve?

A. If your child's asthma is triggered by contact with the cat or when you clean house, you will see some improvement after the cat and the dust are removed. This improvement will increase as the cat dander is removed. However, your child still has overactive airways and may have flares with other triggers.

Q. Do you recommend shots for cat or dog allergies?

A. No, children should avoid cats or dogs if they cause asthma problems.

Q. How frequently do you recommend allergy shots?

A. We recommend immunotherapy for less than five percent of our patients with asthma.

Q. How often are allergy shots given?

A. This can vary considerably. One routine is once or twice a week for the first three to six months, then every one to three weeks.

Q. How many years should a person try the shots before deciding whether to continue or stop?

A. Two years.

NATURAL COURSE

Q. What are the chances that my child will die of asthma?

A. Health statistics show that it is extremely rare for a child to die of asthma in this country. About one hundred deaths are reported annually in children between the ages of one and fifteen years. Put another way, there will be only one death this year for every 25,000 children with asthma. A child with asthma is twice as likely to die in a motor vehicle accident as to die of asthma.

Q. Is it possible for a person's asthma to improve and then to have it recur ten or twenty years later?

A. Yes, about two-thirds of children with asthma improve by the teen years. Much of the improvement may be due to growth in the diameter of their windpipes. Since they do not outgrow their overreactive airways, some of these children may have asthma episodes again later in life.

Q. Is there any way to prevent asthma episodes permanently?

A. No.

Q. Will children who have short flares always continue in this pattern?

A. Each child has an individual pattern or set of patterns. One of my patients has severe three-day flares triggered by contact with a cat and milder two-week flares triggered by a cold.

Q. Do more boys than girls have asthma?

A. Yes, the ratio is about two to one until the teens, when the proportion is even.

Q. Will my child grow out of asthma?

A. A person who has had an asthma episode once has a tendency to have asthma problems in the future. However, growth in the size of the airways makes problems diminish as the child grows from age one year until age five. Many older children also have less trouble as time goes on. The important point is that almost all asthma episodes can be controlled well with a proper treatment plan. Even if your child continues to have asthma problems as a teenager, it should be possible to control them using the proper treatment plan.

Medication

Q. Is it safe to double the dose of medication?

A. Any medication changes should be worked out in advance with your doctor. Ordinarily, doubling the total daily dose of a medication would lead to trouble. The change should be more gradual unless your child has taken the higher dose in the past without problems.

ADRENERGIC DRUGS

Q. How often should you clean an inhaler?

A. A hot water rinse each day of use will keep your inhaler clean. A dirty inhaler will not deliver enough medicine. To check your inhaler, puff it into the air and see if the usual amount of spray is coming out.

Q. Sometimes my child benefits a lot from using the inhaler, other times she seems to get little help, why?

A. The asthma flare may be worse or her technique may be inconsistent. You should check the instructions for inhaler use.

Q. Can you overdose with nebulized medication?

A. I have never seen anyone have toxic effects from using a nebulizer too often. This is because my patients know that if their inhaled medication does not hold them for four hours, it's time to add another drug or to see me. The major problem with frequent use of an inhaler is that the patient is ignoring the fact that asthma is going out of control. That patient can get very, very sick from asthma by not seeking help.

THEOPHYLLINE

Q. What are the long-term adverse effects of theophylline?

A. Although theophylline has been used for decades, physical effects due to long-term use have not been described.

Q. What is a safe and effective theophylline level in the blood?

A. The therapeutic range is between ten and twenty micrograms per milliliter. At a serum concentration of less than five it may not be effective, and over twenty it may cause toxic effects.

Q. Under what circumstances should the level of theophylline in the blood be checked?

A. Child continues to have symptoms on a standard dose.
Dose is increased above usual for age and weight.
There is an increase in adverse effects.
Child takes high doses of theophylline daily.
Child starts taking erythromycin or other drug that increases the theophylline level.

If asthma is well-controlled without adverse effects on standard doses of theophylline, there is no need to check the blood level for the patient with intermittent asthma. Many asthma experts make an annual check on the blood level of a patient who takes theophylline daily.

Q. What purpose does taking less than a "therapeutic dose" of theophylline serve?

A. A lower dose may provide adequate bronchodilation while producing fewer side effects, either when it is used alone or in combination with an adrenergic drug.

Q. What is the best time to get a theophylline level?

A. The best time is approximately three to six hours after the last dose when one is taking a twelve-hour preparation. This will determine the peak level.

STEROIDS

Q. When should a steroid burst be used?

A. Patients taking full doses of bronchodilator drugs (adrenergic alone or adrenergic in combination with theophylline) who continue to have symptoms will benefit from steroid use.

Q. What are the side effects of a steroid burst?

A. When steroids are used for less than two weeks they may cause increased appetite and a good mood.

Q. Is it O.K. for a parent to administer prednisone independently as needed?

A. Yes, but only if you have worked out guidelines for administration with your doctor. It is important to have written guidelines and also a written record of actual use. I have worked out "independent" prednisone use with only two percent of my patients. Another eight percent have a two day supply of prednisone at home but call before using it. The remaining ninety percent are evaluated in the office before treatment with prednisone is considered.

Q. Do steroid bursts lasting from three to seven days cause problems?

A. They have not been shown to cause trouble if they do not occur more than once a month for more than six months in a row. If more frequent bursts are necessary, use of inhaled steroids should be considered.

CROMOLYN

Q. What is the value of cromolyn?

A. On a short-term basis cromolyn blocks the body's reaction to allergens and exercise. On a long-term basis it prevents episodes and thus may reduce or eliminate the need for theophylline or steroids.

Q. Can cromolyn and an adrenergic drug be given simultaneously by compressor-driven nebulizer?

A. Yes. In this case cromolyn takes the place of saline or water.

OTHER MEDICATIONS

Q. Is it safe for my child to take antihistamines? The packages all say they shouldn't be used by a child with asthma.

A. Most asthma experts see no problem with using antihistamines between or during asthma attacks. Antihistamines are prescribed to dry up a post nasal drip that triggers asthma episodes. Theoretically these drugs might dry up the mucus in the windpipes, thus making it harder to cough it up, but this has never been proved.

Q. Can my child use a cough syrup during an attack?

A. In general, it is not a good idea since the cough may be a sign that the asthma is not being adequately treated. Also, the child should be able to cough up the mucus which is blocking the windpipes. However, a cough itself can trigger asthma and sometimes cough medicine is extremely helpful.

Q. What is the effect of the various medications on behavior and moods? Please comment on theophylline, prednisone, metaproterenol, and cromolyn.

A. Theophylline is well known for causing headaches, stomachaches and overactivity. Often this is because the theophylline preparation used causes great fluctuations in serum level during a twelve-hour period. Possible remedies are to change to a theophylline preparation which is released more evenly or to reduce the dose of theophylline.

Prednisone causes an increase in appetite and a good mood in many children just a few days after treatment is started.

Metaproterenol and other beta-adrenergic drugs cause shakiness.

Cromolyn rarely causes significant adverse effects.

Q. Can one build up resistance to asthma medications?

A. Tolerance, or resistance, is a situation in which a given dose of medicine becomes less effective after continued use. The body does not develop tolerance to theophylline, cromolyn, or prednisone. Asthma experts are still debating whether tolerance is a significant problem with respect to adrenergic drugs. It has not been a problem for our patients.

Home Treatment

Q. When should I start giving medication?

A. Ordinarily you should start treatment according to a prearranged plan as soon as you recognize the first sign of asthma in your child. For some, there is an early clue such as an itch on the neck, a sneeze or a runny nose. For others a cough, a wheeze or tight chest is the first sign of asthma. For children four years and over, use the peak flow reading as your guide.

Q. Why does my child have a flare when he is already taking medication?

A. The dose of medication that controls a flare provoked by one trigger may not be adequate when another trigger is added to the system. A single drug may control an episode that was triggered by an upper respiratory infection. Additional triggers such as cold air, an allergen or exercise might produce further reaction in the bronchioles which cannot be contained by the original dose of medication.

Q. How can dosage of medication be determined without frequent phone calls or visits to the doctor?

A. You and your doctor should work out a plan in advance that covers the various possibilities that may occur. This could be based on medication routines that are described in chapter four.

Q. How long after symptoms subside should medicine be taken?

A. Usually it's a good idea to continue the full dose of medication until there have been no symptoms, or until peak flow has been in the green zone for two days, before beginning to taper. See Medication Routines in chapter four.

Q. Should I start giving my child medicine at the onset of a cold?

A. If your child develops asthma symptoms with most colds or upper respiratory infections, it would make a lot of sense to start treating with asthma medications at the onset of a cold. You should work out a plan with your physician so that you are prepared.

Q. What type of patient should use a holding chamber to deliver inhaled medications?

A. Almost every patient will benefit from using a holding chamber with an MDI. Some patients can substitute this method for treatment with a compressor-driven nebulizer.

Q. Should every child with asthma use a peak flow meter at home?

A. Most children age four years and over will benefit from use of the peak flow meter at home—both to learn about asthma and to regulate medication use. A peak flow whistle can be used for two- and three-year-olds.

Q. Does peak flow vary with age?

A. Yes, but height is the major variable in children.

Q. Under what circumstances should I come to see the doctor?

A. If you cannot judge how your child is doing during an episode , you should see the doctor. You should work out a plan of treatment for the present episode. At a follow-up visit, make sure you work out a written plan for future episodes. Don't go just for treatment. Make sure you learn something at every visit.

Q. How often should I visit the doctor if I know the four signs of asthma trouble and can manage attacks at home?

A. After an initial period during which we work out a treatment plan, my patients come in every three to twelve months.

Q. Why does asthma worsen after finishing medication?

A. If an asthma episode worsens after medication is stopped, it means that the changes in the bronchioles have not yet cleared up. Medication will have to be resumed.

Q. How long should or does an asthma episode last?

A. The duration of an asthma episode is extremely variable—lasting from hours to many days. With prompt and proper treatment, symptoms should improve dramatically within a period of hours.

Q. Do children take medicine all year long?

A. Some take it every day, some half the time, and others only for a total of a few days or weeks per year.

Q. How much should a child with asthma drink during an asthma episode?

A. In general, we recommend the usual body requirement for size if there is no fever. This is 32 ounces for a child who weighs thirty pounds and 64 ounces for a child who weighs ninety pounds or over.

Families and Asthma

Q. How do you get teenagers to take medications that cause headache and stomach ache?

A. The teenager will decide whether medication side effects are preferable to an episode. Remember that adverse effects can be reduced by taking a smaller dose of medicine. There are several medications to choose from. If one is unacceptable, another should be tried.

Q. How can I get my daughter to help herself?

A. Two-year-olds have learned to tell their parents when they aren't feeling well. Most three-year-olds can use an inhaler with a reservoir if they have adequate coordination and are properly motivated and trained. Some ten-year-olds can judge their symptoms and take their medications without direct supervision. The child who does not cooperate in the treatment of her asthma does not understand her responsibility in the treatment process. She probably feels that she cannot control her asthma and is angry when other people try to do it for her. She should read the book *Teaching Myself About Asthma* and decide with her parents what responsibility she will take on and what part of it is theirs.

Q. How do you get a teenager to take medication regularly?

A. In general, the asthma management schedule should be worked out by the doctor and older teenagers. Their tasks should be clear. They should realize that if they skip their medication or come in contact with an allergen, they will probably have an asthma flare. After a couple of episodes, most teenagers figure out what they can do to cut down on frequency and severity. If a teenager doesn't want to take medicine, bugging is pointless. An attack can be a good learning experience in these situations. It is a good idea for young teens to take over most of the responsibility for their asthma. This is not always possible.

Q. How responsible are teenagers for taking care of their asthma?

A. Most teenagers in my practice do an excellent job in managing their asthma. Sometimes they consult with their parents for advice. At other times they check with me. Friends of one of my patients who plays varsity basketball make her use her inhaler before each game. They know she will play better and they want their team to win.

Q. How do you deal with the feeling of being different?

A. People with asthma are different—in one way. They have overactive airways. Most of the "feeling different" that I have seen has been inflicted by well-meaning doctors, teachers or parents. Children with asthma can play all sports and take part in all physical activities no matter how strenuous, unless they are in the middle of an episode. Less than two percent of our patients have to watch their activity closely between episodes.

Q. What do you think of exercise programs for children with asthma?

A. A child with asthma that is well-controlled will be able to take part in any exercise or sports program and does not need a special routine.

Q. Can you suggest a diet to control asthma?

A. Any well-balanced diet would be satisfactory unless the child has food allergies.

Q. Should I allow my son to stay at a friend's house if I know it will trigger an asthma episode?

A. The two things we should know before answering are: How bad are the episodes? Certainly a serious attack that causes your son to miss school and to require a doctor's assistance should be avoided. Can the episode be prevented by taking medication before and during the visit? If so, it is reasonable to permit the visit.

Q. How can the child learn to take care of herself?

A. Children learn one step at a time. First they have to be able to recognize the earliest sign of asthma. Then they should learn what to do, depending on their age: tell a parent, avoid the trigger, take medicine, and drink warm liquid.

Q. What is the effect on other children in the family when attention is showered on the child with asthma?

A. Usually not good. Parenting is always a balancing act. It is important to see that everyone in the family receives a fair share of attention.

Q. What should you do when you sense that your child feels like a nuisance to friends or their families?

A. Plan how to intervene in an asthma flare. Encourage your child to take as much responsibility as possible for each episode. The responsible child is less likely to feel like a nuisance than the helpless child.

School and Travel

Q. What should I do when traveling?

A. You should have a travel check list. Take your instructions, Asthma Record, and Emergency Room Doctor Letter with you, as well as an adequate supply of all your child's medicines (properly labeled). If your child gets into trouble from contact with cats, pre-treat before contact. It is better to start too early than too late. If possible, call your own doctor for advice before going to the emergency room.

Q. Why does asthma occur at the most inopportune times?

A. There is an asthma rule which states, "If something is going to go wrong, it will be at an inconvenient time." The logic goes as follows: When you are relaxed and well organized, it is possible to keep track of three medications, exposure to cats and cigarette smoke and to see that your child gets adequate rest. If there is a disruption in your pattern of living because of illness, traveling, a wedding, or the arrival of visitors for the weekend, it is harder to follow the usual routine and to notice the early signs of an asthma flare.

Q. My son starts nursery school this fall. He has severe asthma. How do we deal with the school?

A. You should give the teachers or school nurse a copy of *Children With Asthma: A Manual For Parents* and request that they read Basic Facts. In addition, you should provide them with specific information about your child by completing the Forms for Teacher and for School Nurse to be found in chapter six. Finally, you should offer to meet with them to discuss any questions they might have about your child's health, activity, or behavior at school.

How to Improve Your Child's Care

Q. When will I be able to handle an episode properly?

A. If you can answer all the questions on the Asthma Quiz (chapter four) and have kept accurate records of your observations for two or three episodes, you should be able to handle most of them at home.

Q. Where can you buy a peak flow meter?

A. See Resource section, p. 248.

Q. Please outline a reasonable plan for treating an asthma attack.

A. First, eliminate triggers, then assess severity of episode, give medicines, limit activity, and consult doctor if not improving as expected.

Resource List

Books

Asthma: The Complete Guide To Self-Management Of Asthma And Allergies For Patients And Their Families
A. M. Weinstein, M.D.
350 pages, $17.95.
McGraw-Hill, 1987.

This excellent book focuses on the problems of adults. The basics of asthma and allergies and the medications used to treat them are described in a clear fashion. Dr. Weinstein includes eleven sample programs for managing mild, moderate, and severe asthma. There is a seventeen-page chapter on children with asthma.

Living With Asthma
Part 1: Manual for teaching parents the self-management of childhood asthma. Part 2: Manual for teaching children the self-management of asthma.
Thomas L. Creer
773 pages, 1986, $40.00.
The Asthma Project, Attn. Christine Krutzsch
National Heart, Lung, and Blood Institute
NIH Building 31, Room 4A–21
Bethesda, MD 20092
(301) 496–4236

This outstanding resource for parents' support groups provides accurate information, illustrations, and handouts for parents. Detailed instructions guide the leader through two sessions on the basics of asthma and medications. Six sessions provide extensive discussion of the early warning signs and triggers of asthma, positive reinforcement of desired behavior and problem-solving techniques. The second volume is designed for a concurrent children's program.

Luke Has Asthma Too
A. Rogers
32 pages, illustrated, 1987, $6.95.
Waterfront Books
98 Brookes Avenue
Burlington, VT 05401

This book will make for good reading with your child whether or not he or she has asthma. The narrative conveys the feeling that asthma can be managed in a calm fashion. This is an important message for the more than two million families that have children with asthma.

Manual Of Problems In Asthma, Allergy And Related Disorders
D. Bukstein, and R. Strunk, eds.
293 pages, $18.95.
Little, Brown and Co., 1984.

A collection of short, sophisticated summaries of common clinical problems in asthma and allergy. Covers triggers, infections, psychological considerations, exercise-induced asthma, pregnancy, surgery, as well as excellent descriptions of the common drugs used to treat asthma. An annotated list of medical references accompanies each section.

Peak Performance: A Strategy for Asthma Self Assessment
G. Mendoza
64 pages, $10.00
Order from:
Mothers of Asthmatics, Inc.
5316 Summit Drive
Fairfax, VA 22030

A helpful guide to peak flow monitoring for physicians, parents and patients.

Teaching Myself About Asthma
G. Parcel, K. Tiernan, P. Nader, and L. Weiner
152 pages, 250 illustrations by Mark Weakley, 1984, $9.95.
Health Education Associates
14 North Lake Road
Columbia, SC 29223

Clearly written and well-illustrated, this workbook is geared to the reading abilities of children nine to twelve years of age. Learning activities are suggested which demonstrate the basics of breathing, the causes, prevention, and treatment of asthma, and the child's role in its management. Parent and child can read the book together.

Newsletters

Asthma Update
David Jamison, Editor
123 Monticello Avenue
Annapolis, MD 21401

Quarterly newsletter for parents and adult patients. Includes annotated abstracts from current medical journals and perspectives on asthma by health professionals. Four to six pages per issue. $8.00 per year.

MA Report
Nancy Sander, Editor
5316 Summit Drive
Fairfax, VA 22030
(703) 631–0123

"A support system in a newsletter" published by Mothers of Asthmatics, Inc. Practical and positive information for parents of asthmatic children. $10 for 12 monthly issues.

Video Tapes

Asthma and Allergies in the School: The Importance of Cooperative Care
Twelve minutes
Parents, children, and teachers talk about managing asthma and allergies in school. Supplementary written material available for parents and teachers.

For free loan video, write to:
    Modern Talking Pictures
    5000 Park Street North
    St. Petersburg, FL 33709
    (813) 541–5763

You Can Control Asthma
Fifteen minutes
Lively discussion of asthma triggers, warning signs and taking medicine.

Written guidelines for a nurse educator and materials for patients and parents. Write:

Virginia Taggart, MPH
Georgetown CIRID
Department of Community and Family Medicine
Georgetown University Medical School
3900 Reservoir Road NW
Washington, DC 20007
(202) 687–1611

Organizations

American Lung Association
1740 Broadway
New York, NY 10019

The more than 300 local and state lung assocations provide many asthma education services including family asthma programs and "Super Stuff." Some chapters sponsor support groups and newsletters. Local affiliates are listed in the white pages under Lung Assocation.

American Academy of Allergy and Immunology
611 East Wells Street
Milwaukee, WI 53202
(414) 272–6071

Pamphlets on asthma, allergies, mold and pollen.

Asthma and Allergy Foundation of America
1717 Massachusetts Avenue
Washington, DC 20036
(202) 265–0265

A number of chapters throughout the country offer support groups, school programs, community workshops and conferences.

Asthma Consultants
125 Red Gate Lane
Amherst, MA 01002

Offers consultation service for health maintenance organizations, group practices, hospitals, support groups, and governmental bodies committed to improving the care of children with asthma.

Mothers of Asthmatics, Inc.
5316 Summit Drive
Fairfax, VA 22030
(703) 631–0123

Nonprofit organization provides support for the parents of asthmatic children through *MA Report,* a newsletter; *Team Work,* an annual resource list which includes publications, organizations, vendors, camps; and other creative links with parents of children with asthma.

National Foundation for Asthma
Tucson Medical Center
P.O. Box 30069
Tucson, AZ 85751–0069
(602) 323–6046

Free pamphlets: "Asthma: Fact & Fiction", "Dust 'N Stuff", and "Weeds 'N Things."

National Heart, Lung, and Blood Institute
NIH Building 31, Room 4A–21
9000 Rockville Pike
Bethesda, MD 20892
(301) 496–4236

Free fourteen-page "Asthma Reading and Resource List." Four educational programs for parents and children. "Living with Asthma," "Open Airways," "Air Power," and "Air Wise," teach basic skills. These include recognizing early signs, identifying and controlling triggers, attack management steps, taking meds properly, coping skills, and improving communication with your doctor.

National Institute of Allergy and Infectious Diseases
NIH Building 31, Room 7A–32
9000 Rockville Pike
Bethesda, MD 20892
(301) 496–4000

Informative free pamphlets on dust allergy, mold allergy, pollen allergy and sinusitis.

National Jewish Center for Immunology and Respiratory Disease
1400 Jackson Street
Denver, CO 80206
(800) 222–LUNG

Provides information on asthma and lung disease via the toll-free LUNG LINE, (800) 222–LUNG. Engaged in treatment, research and education in chronic respiratory diseases. Accepts patients through physician referral.

Equipment Vendors

Allergy Control Products
89 Danbury Road, P.O. Box 793
Ridgefield, CT 06877
(in CT call 1–483–9580)
(800) 422–DUST

High quality dust-proof encasings and room air cleaners. Free information sheets on dust and mold control.

Bio-Tech Systems
P.O. Box 25380
Chicago, IL 60625
(312) 465–8020
(800) 621–5545

Distributors of allergy, asthma, and respiratory supplies.

Biotrine Corporation
52 Dragon Court
Woburn, MA 01801
(617) 935–8844

Peak flow monitor (whistle).

Clement Clarke, Inc.
3128 East 17 Avenue
 Suite C and D
Columbus, Ohio 43219
(800) 848–8923

Mini-Wright peak flow meter.
Low-range Mini-Wright peak flow meter.

Devilbiss Company
P.O. Box 835
Somerset, PA 15501
(814) 443–4881

Pulmo-Aide compressor-driven nebulizer.

Healthscan Products, Inc.
908 Pompton Avenue
Cedar Grove, NJ 07009
(201) 857-3414
(800) 962-1266

Assess peak flow meter.

Key Pharmaceuticals, Inc.
2000 Galloping Hill Road
Kenilworth, NJ 07033
(201) 298-4000

InspirEase and INHAL-AID holding chambers.

Monaghan Medical Corporation
P.O. Box 978
Plattsburgh, NY 12901
(518) 561-7330
(800) 833-9653

AeroChamber holding chamber.

Mountain Medical Equipment, Inc.
10488 West Centennial Road
Littleton, CO 80127
(303) 973-1200
(800) 525-8950

Medi-Mist compressor-driven nebulizer.

Medical Bibliography

Articles

Bernstein, I. Leonard. 1985. Cromolyn Sodium in the Treatment of Asthma: Coming of Age in the United States. *Journal of Allergy and Clinical Immunology.* 76:381–88.

Brunette, Michele G., Larry Lands and Louis-Phillipe Thibodeau. 1988. Childhood Asthma: Prevention of Attacks with Short-Term Corticosteroid Treatment of Upper Respiratory Tract Infection. *Pediatrics* 81:624–629.

Burrows, Benjamin. 1987. The Natural History of Asthma. *Journal of Allergy and Clinical Immunology.* 80:373–77.

Harper, Thomas B., and Robert Strunk. 1981. Techniques of Administration of Metered-Dose Aerosolized Drugs in Asthmatic Children. *American Journal of Diseases of Childhood.* 135:218–21.

Harris, James B., Miles M. Weinberger, Edward Nassif, Gary Smith, Gary Milavetz, and Allan Stillerman. 1987. Early Intervention with Short Courses of Prednisone to Prevent Progression of Asthma in Ambulatory Patients Incompletely Responsive to Bronchodilators. *Journal of Pediatrics.* 110:627–33.

Hendeles, Leslie, and Miles M. Weinberger. 1986. Selection of a Slow-Release Theophylline Product. *Journal of Allergy and Clinical Immunology.* 78:743–51.

Hilman, B. C., L. Bairnsfather, W. Washburne, and A. L. Vekovius. 1987. Nebulized Cromolyn Sodium: Safety, Efficacy, and Role in the Management of Childhood Asthma. *Pediatric Asthma, Allergy and Immunology.* 1:43–52.

251

Hsu, Katherine H. K., Daniel E. Jenkins, Bartholomew P. Hsi, Erwin Bourhofer, Virginia Thompson, Frank C. F. Hsu, and Susan C. Jacob. 1979. Ventilatory Functions of Normal Children and Young Adults— Mexican-American, White, and Black. *Journal of Pediatrics.* 95:192–96.

Iafrate, R. Peter, Kenneth L. Massey, and Leslie Hendeles. 1986. Current Concepts in Clinical Therapeutics: Asthma. *Clinical Pharmacy.* 5:206–27.

Levison, H., P. A. Reilly, and G. H. Worsley. 1985. Spacing Devices and Metered-Dose Inhalers in Childhood Asthma. *Journal of Pediatrics.* 107:662–68.

McFadden, E. R., Jr. 1985. Clinical Use of Beta-Adrenergic Agonists. *Journal of Allergy and Clinical Immunology.* 76:352–56.

Nelson, Harold S. 1986. Adrenergic Therapy of Bronchial Asthma. *Journal of Allergy and Clinical Immunology.* 77:771–85.

Newhouse, Michael T., and Myrna B. Dolovich. 1986. Control of Asthma by Aerosols. *New England Journal of Medicine.* 315:870–74.

Robertson, Colin F., Freda Smith, Raphael Beck, and Henry Levison. 1985. Response to Frequent Low Dose of Nebulized Salbutamol in Acute Asthma. *Journal of Pediatrics.* 106:672–74.

Selcow, Jay E., L. Mendelson, J. P. Rosen. 1983. A Comparison of Cromolyn and Bronchodilators in Patients with Mild to Moderately Severe Asthma in an Office Practice. *Annals of Allergy.* 50:13–18.

Siegel, Sheldon C. 1985. Overview of Corticosteroid Therapy. *Journal of Allergy and Clinical Immunology.* 76:312–20.

Williams, M. Henry, Jr. 1982. Expiratory Flow Rates: Their Role in Asthma Therapy. *Hospital Practice.* 17:95–110

Drugs for Asthma. *Medical Letter* (1987) 29:11–16

Books

Bierman, C. Warren, and David S. Pearlman, eds. *Allergic Diseases of Infancy, Childhood and Adolescence.* Philadelphia: W. B. Saunders Company, 1980.

Bukstein, Donald, and Robert Strunk, eds. *Manual of Problems in Asthma, Allergy, and Related Disorders.* Boston: Little, Brown and Co., 1984.

Kendig, Edwin L., and Victor Chernick, eds. *Disorders of the Respiratory Tract in Children.* Philadelphia: W. B. Saunders Company, 1983.

Middleton, Elliot, Charles E. Reed, Elliot F. Ellis, N. Franklin Adkinson, Jr. and John W. Yunginger, eds. *Allergy: Principles and Practice.* 2 vols. St. Louis: The C. V. Mosby Company, 1988.

Tinkelman, David G., Constantine J. Falliers, and Charles K. Naspitz, eds. *Childhood Asthma Pathophysiology and Treatment.* New York: Marcel Dekker, Inc., 1987.

United States Pharmacopeial Convention, Inc., eds. *USPDI: Drug Information for the Health Care Provider.* Rockville, MD, 1987.

Food and Drug Administration Approval of Drugs

Congress mandated the Food and Drug Administration (FDA) to regulate the evaluation, manufacture, distribution, labeling and advertising of prescription drugs. Under FDA regulations, drug manufacturers must conduct clinical trials to document the safety and effectiveness of new drugs for specific uses. These trials produce data based on the age of the patients as well as on the dose and the route of administration of the drug. The FDA staff then evaluates these data.

Manufacturers have not yet supplied the FDA with enough data on some drugs to determine whether they are safe and effective in young children. Thus, some asthma drugs carry the statement, "the safety and effectiveness in children under [number] years of age have not been established for this product." None of the four drug formulations I use most often in the treatment of asthma in children *under the age of two years* has been found to be safe and effective in this age group by the FDA. This does not mean that these drugs are dangerous, only that sufficient data to establish their safety and effectiveness in children have not been forwarded to the FDA.

The FDA commented on this situation in *The FDA Drug Bulletin,* of April 1982, as follows:

Use of Approved Drugs for Unlabeled Indications

The appropriateness or the legality of prescribing approved drugs for uses not included in their official labeling is sometimes a cause of concern and confusion among practitioners.

Under the Federal Food, Drug, and Cosmetic (FD&C) Act, a drug approved for marketing may be labeled, promoted, and advertised by the manufacturer only for those uses for which the drug's safety and effectiveness have been established and which FDA has approved. These are commonly referred to as "approved uses." This means that adequate and well-controlled clinical trials have documented these uses, and the results of the trials have been reviewed and approved by FDA.

The FD&C Act does not, however, limit the manner in which a physician may use an approved drug. Once a product has been approved for marketing, a physician may prescribe it for uses or in treatment regimens or patient populations that are not included in approved labeling. *Such "unapproved" or, more precisely, "unlabeled" uses may be appropriate and rational in certain circumstances, and may, in fact, reflect approaches to drug therapy that have been extensively reported in medical literature.*

The term "unapproved uses" is, to some extent, misleading. It includes a variety of situations ranging from unstudied to thoroughly investigated drug uses. Valid new uses for drugs already on the market are often first discovered through serendipitous observations and therapeutic innovations, subsequently confirmed by well-planned and executed clinical investigations. Before such advances can be added to the approved labeling, however, data substantiating the effectiveness of a new use or regimen must be submitted by the manufacturer to FDA for evaluation. This may take time and, without the initiative of the drug manufacturer whose product is involved, may never occur. For that reason, *accepted medical practice often includes drug use that is not reflected in approved drug labeling* (italics mine).

The prescription of a drug for a condition or an age group not included on the label is entirely proper if it is based on "rational scientific theory, reliable medical opinion, or controlled clinical studies" according to *AMA Drug Evaluations* published in 1986. Medical journals frequently contain studies that report on the effectiveness of old drugs for new uses or new techniques for using an old drug. The FDA does not revise its assessment of drugs to include new uses or techniques of administration unless a drug company or other interested party requests a change and supplies the necessary data. Often no such request is made.

The laws under which the FDA operates have protected the American people from using inadequately tested drugs. However, every drug, whether approved by the FDA or not, can cause adverse effects. Physicians and parents share the responsibility of monitoring children with asthma carefully and in a timely manner to be sure that each drug is having the intended beneficial effect and not causing serious adverse effects.

Glossary

acceptance:
: agreeing to a treatment routine based on understanding

Accurbron:
: a brand name for theophylline

acute:
: comes on suddenly

adrenalin:
: an adrenergic drug produced by the body; same as epinephrine

adrenergic:
: adrenalin-type drug

adverse:
: undesirable

AeroBid:
: a brand name for flunisolide, an aerosol steroid preparation

albuterol:
: beta-adrenergic drug

allergen:
: any substance that causes the manifestations of allergy

Alupent:
: a brand name for metaproterenol

alveoli:
: air sacs located at the end of the tiniest bronchioles

antibody:
: protein which develops in response to a foreign substance (antigen)

antihistamine:
: a class of drug that blocks the actions of histamine such as swelling and itching

asymptomatic:
: without symptoms

asthma:
: reversible obstructive airway disease

attack:
: a dramatic word for an episode or flare of asthma

Azmacort:
: a brand name for triamcinolone, an aerosol steroid preparation

beclomethasone:	an aerosol steroid drug
Beclovent:	a brand name for beclomethasone, an aerosol steroid preparation
book:	to leave quickly
Brethaire:	a brand name for terbutaline, an aerosol preparation
Brethine:	a brand name for terbutaline, an aerosol preparation
Bricanyl:	a brand name for terbutaline
bronchi:	large air passages or windpipes
bronchioles:	smaller air passages or windpipes
bronchiolitis:	inflammation, caused by a virus, of the smallest bronchioles
bronchitis:	inflammation of the bronchi
bronchoconstriction:	narrowing of the bronchioles; opposite of bronchodilation
bronchodilator:	a drug which causes the bronchioles to open
bronchospasm:	tightening of the muscles around the airways, making them narrow
capillary:	tiniest blood vessels
cartilage:	dense tissue which girds the large airways
cc:	abbreviation for cubic centimeter; equivalent to a milliliter or 1/1000 of a liter. This metric measure is equal to 1/5 of a measuring teaspoon.
chronic:	continuous or long-term
cilia:	tiny hair-like processes which project from the surface of the cells which line the airway
compliance:	doing exactly what your doctor says whether or not you understand it
controlled-release:	same as long-acting, sustained-release, slow-release
corticosteroid:	another term for steroid or cortisone-like drug
coughing asthma:	a form of asthma in which coughing is the only symptom and there is no abnormality in any lung function test
cromolyn:	drug which prevents degranulation of mast cells and thus prevents an asthma attack

croup:
illness in which the larynx and trachea are inflamed. Usually caused by a virus; produces a barking cough.

dander:
scales of dead skin

decaliter:
1/10 of a liter

eczema:
a skin rash also known as atopic dermatitis

Elixophyllin:
a brand name for theophylline

episode:
synonymous with attack or flare

exacerbation:
worsening

exercise-induced asthma:
a form of asthma in which exercise is the only trigger

exhale:
to breathe out

expiration:
act of breathing out

fast-release:
synonymous with plain or regular when referring to theophylline preparation

flare:
synonymous with attack or episode

flunisolide:
an aerosol steroid drug

gastroesophageal reflux:
backward flow of material from stomach to esophagus. Causes irritation which can lead to bronchospasm.

Gyrocaps:
Slophyllin slow-release capsule

HEPA filter:
abbreviation for high efficiency particulate air filter; removes tiny particles from the air

hives:
itchy swellings of skin usually due to allergy

holding chamber:
a device which holds mist produced by metered-dose inhaler. Also known as extender, reservoir or spacer.

hydrocortisone:
a steroid drug

hyperventilation:
excessive rate and depth of breathing

IgE:
immunoglobulin gamma E. Production of this antibody is often provoked by allergens

immunotherapy:
synonymous with allergy shots, injection treatment, hypo-sensitization, desensitization

indication:
reason to use

inhaler:	also metered-dose inhaler (MDI), device for creating a mist of drug which can be drawn directly into the windpipes

I/O ratio:	relative length of inspiration compared to expiration (same as I/E ratio)

inspiration:	act of breathing in

inspiration-expiration ratio:
	same as I/O ratio

Intal:	a brand name for cromolyn

intradermal:	into the skin

intravenous:	into the vein

irritant:	a non-allergenic substance which may provoke a reaction in the airways

kg:	kilogram, 1,000 grams or 2.2 pounds

liter:	metric measurement, slightly more than a quart

long-acting:	synonymous with slow-release or sustained-release, refers to theophylline preparation

maintenance medication:
	a drug given on a regular basis to help prevent symptoms

mast cell:	one of the cell types which contain chemicals that can produce the asthma reaction

mcg:	microgram, 1/1,000,000 of a gram

MDI:	metered-dose inhaler

mean peak flow rate:
	the average of the highest expiratory rates for a group children of a certain height expressed in liters per minute

mediator:	a chemical which is the "middle man" in a physiological reaction

metabolize:	to change chemically or physically

Metaprel:	a brand name for metaproterenol

metaproterenol:	an adrenergic drug

methylprednisolone: a steroid drug

mg:	milligram, 1/1000 of a gram
mite:	tiny arachnid found in house dust; may cause allergic asthma
ml:	milliliter, 1/1,000 of a liter, same as a cc
mucus:	protective and cleansing material produced by glands in the bronchioles
nebulizer:	a device which converts liquid into a spray
para-nasal sinuses:	one of the four bone-enclosed cavities surrounding the nose
peak flow meter:	a device used to measure peak expiratory flow rate
peak flow rate:	actual highest expiratory flow rate
pollen:	microspores of a seed plant
pollutant:	an impurity
prednisone:	a steroid drug
prednisolone:	a steroid drug
prick test:	type of skin test for allergy
Proventil:	a brand name for albuterol
pulmonary function test:	
	a test or series of tests used to measure various aspects of lung function and capacity
Quibron T/SR:	a brand name for theophylline
retraction:	a sucking in of the chest skin
ROAD:	reversible obstructive airway disease
score:	peak flow meter reading expressed in liters per minute
serum:	the liquid portion of the blood
side effect:	undesired or adverse effect of drug
sinusitis:	inflammation of one or more para-nasal sinuses
Slo-bid:	a brand name for a theophylline preparation
Slo-Phyllin:	a brand name for a theophylline preparation
Somophyllin:	a brand name for a theophylline preparation
Spinhaler:	a device for delivering cromolyn sodium

steroids:	a type of hormone produced by the adrenal cortex
subcutaneous:	under the skin
sustained-release:	synonymous with long-acting or slow-release, refers to theophylline preparation
sympathomimetic:	produces same effect as epinephrine injection or stimulation of sympathetic nervous system
Theo-Dur:	brand name for a long-acting theophylline preparation
terbutaline:	an adrenergic drug
theophylline:	a commonly used bronchodilator
toxicity:	quality of being poisonous; the adverse effect(s) of a drug
triamcinolone:	a steroid drug
trigger:	instigator, precipitating factor
twitchy:	overreactive
Vanceril:	a brand name for beclomethasone
Ventolin:	a brand name for albuterol
wheeze:	high pitched whistling which occurs when air flows through narrowed bronchial tube
work-up:	evaluation of a patient

Index

Page numbers in bold face refer to illustrations.

Order Form

You should be able to buy *Children With Asthma: A Manual For Parents* at any bookstore. If this is not possible, please use this form.

Pedipress, Inc.
125 Red Gate Lane
Amherst, MA 01002

Please send _____ copies of *Children With Asthma: A Manual For Parents* at $11.95 plus $1.00 postage—**$12.95 per book.**

Name: _____

Address: _____

_____ Zip: _____

In Massachusetts: please add sixty cents sales tax for each book.

Air Mail or United Parcel Service—**$13.95 per book.**

Send check or money order. No cash or C.O.D.s please.

Order Form

You should be able to buy *Children With Asthma: A Manual For Parents* at any bookstore. If this is not possible, please use this form.

Pedipress, Inc.
125 Red Gate Lane
Amherst, MA 01002

Please send _____ copies of *Children With Asthma: A Manual For Parents* at $11.95 plus $1.00 postage—**$12.95 per book.**

Name: _____

Address: _____

_____ Zip: _____

In Massachusetts: please add sixty cents sales tax for each book.

Air Mail or United Parcel Service—**$13.95 per book.**

Send check or money order. No cash or C.O.D.s please.